R2004221e7248

MECHANICSVILLE BRANCH
ATLANTA-FULTON PUBLIC LIBRARY SYSTEM
400 FORMWAL STREET SW
ATLANTA, GEORGIA 30312

Praise for *Stay, Breathe with Me: The Gift of Compassionate Medicine*

W9-BXN-054

"Unlike much of medical literature, even in the area of death and dying, this volume by Helen Allison and Irene Allison is written from the heart and speaks to the heart. Therein lies its transformative power. As a former palliative care physician and future dying human, I am profoundly grateful."

—**Gabor Maté, MD,** best-selling author of *When The Body Says No: The Cost of Hidden Stress*

"I hope this deeply compassionate, wise and enchanting book will be widely read by those who work in 'mainstream' medicine, and not just palliative care. We forget that suffering is often the cause and not just the result of illness. Palliative care, with its focus on the alleviation of suffering and the healing power of compassion, has so much to teach modern medicine. The best lessons in this wonderful book are the stories of what went wrong: with deep humanity the authors lead us through loss and confusion to places of love, wisdom and healing. So many health professionals need this understanding and healing in their own lives."

—**Robin Youngson, MD,** co-founder of Hearts in Healthcare, author of *Time to Care: How to Love your Patients and your Job*

"It is a privilege to recommend this book to doctors, nurses, social workers, and other practitioners of the healing arts as they try to improve their skills at treating the chronically and terminally ill. Others interested in how best to approach such patients will find it a wonderful read."

—**Lawrence P. Levitt, MD,** Professor of Clinical Medicine, Penn State College of Medicine; Senior Consultant, Neurology Emeritus, Lehigh Valley Hospital; coauthor of *Uncommon Wisdom: True Tales of What Our Lives as Doctors Have Taught Us about Love, Faith, and Healing*

"Beautifully and tenderly written … the gentle weaving of these stories reminds us to mix equal parts of technology, love, and compassion throughout our lives to the end … for all caregivers, these stories underline the need for technology to be wedded to love and compassion at the end of life."

—**Carol McVeigh, RN,** Palliative Care Nurse, Canada (1943–2015)

"*Stay, Breath with Me* is a passionate, heartfelt plea for medicine to return to the practice of compassion and empathy. It's an antidote to the over-medicalization of medicine, particularly when it comes to end-of life care. Irene and Helen Allison seek our thoughtful consideration—through a number of touching case studies—and demonstrate how palliative care can ease dying. This book is an important contribution to the growing discussion on how we die today. I hope its wisdom influences current and future generations of physicians, nurses and caregivers."

—**Phil Dwyer,** author, *Conversations On Dying*

"Compelling reading for families of persons with life-threatening illnesses and their healthcare professionals. Many people back away from living with death as one's constant companion. This book permits us to envision living with dying in a humane, compassionate manner."

—**Mary Valentich, PhD**, Professor Emerita, Faculty of Social Work, University of Calgary, Canada

"Helen Allison, a compassionate, caring nurse with a special insight into the feelings of patients in pain and a nurse who must have been loved and respected by patients and peers. This book is a must read for all health care professionals."

—**Rhoda Anderson**, President, Lakes District Unit, Canadian Cancer Society, Hospice Volunteer, Canada

"In some ways I know much more than I knew when I first started at St. Paul's Palliative Care Unit, and in other ways there is so much I don't know and don't have the skills or wisdom to address, and those are the issues that you particularly address—namely, suffering, the relief of suffering, and meaning—meaning of the illness, and meaning of one's life, particularly if life is seen to be in jeopardy. Your stories/vignettes take us to the places where we feel uncomfortable and where we fear to go, but where we do need to go, particularly if we [are to] do more than just lip service to the concept of true, holistic palliative care."

—**Millie Cumming-Chalmers, MD**, Palliative Care Physician, Canada

"Helen Allison, the first palliative care head nurse at St. Boniface in Winnipeg, knows and practices the philosophy that caring endures when curing is no longer possible. Her stories, which are filled with compassion, empathy and wisdom, are heartwarming and instructive."

—**Sandra Martin,** The Long Goodbye columnist, The Globe and Mail, author of *A Good Death: Making the Most of our Final Choices*

Stay, Breathe with Me

The Gift of
Compassionate Medicine

Helen Allison, RN, MSW

with Irene Allison

Foreword by Dr. Rev. David Skelton

SHE WRITES PRESS

Copyright © 2016 by Helen Allison and Irene Allison

All rights reserved. No part of this publication may be reproduced, distributed, or transmitted in any form or by any means, including photocopying, recording, digital scanning, or other electronic or mechanical methods, without the prior written permission of the publisher, except in the case of brief quotations embodied in critical reviews and certain other noncommercial uses permitted by copyright law. For permission requests, please address She Writes Press.

Published 2016
Printed in the United States of America
ISBN: 978-1-63152-062-4
Library of Congress Control Number: 2015960992

Cover design by Rebecca Lown
Interior design by Tabitha Lahr

For information, address:
She Writes Press
1563 Solano Ave #546
Berkeley, CA 94707

She Writes Press is a division of SparkPoint Studio, LLC.

In loving memory of my daughter,
Leslie Allison (1952–2010)

"Music for a while shall all your cares beguile . . ."
—Henry Purcell (1659–1695)

Leslie's love of music, its meaning, and its enchantment were the essence of her life. International acclaim as a soprano is the gift she leaves behind. Irreversible illness and surgery left her paralyzed and impaired her speech. When professional caregivers drowned her whispering, faltering voice, Leslie suffered disparity and despair. She had lost her sense of self. For there was no narrative, no dialog to relieve the chaos of ungoverned thoughts that occupied her mind.

And yet my daughter grew in stature from the suffering she endured. The music that she loved became the parable, or story, of her journey through illness. She found comfort in the knowledge that music needs no words to inspire courage, joy, and hope. Music is the universal language of the soul, crossing cultural boundaries to reach us all.

So Leslie began to hum. Humming released her from the tyranny of fear, and loss of dignity and self-respect. And oh what joy she knew when she rediscovered her singing voice. The melodic harmony of humming comforted her body, mind, and soul. From behind her illness, the person who was Leslie reemerged.

My daughter never regained her ability to walk. Yet Leslie's indomitable spirit survived. Despite her serious illness, she pursued her university studies and obtained her master of arts degree. And, confined to her wheelchair, she performed several concerts for charity. To those in need, Leslie's gift of music inspired dignity and hope. Towards the end of Leslie's life, Nurse Bonnie gently affirmed, "I love it when Leslie hums and sings."

The echo of my daughter's voice lives within the pages of this book. She walked the way of those who suffer to offer tender compassion and care.

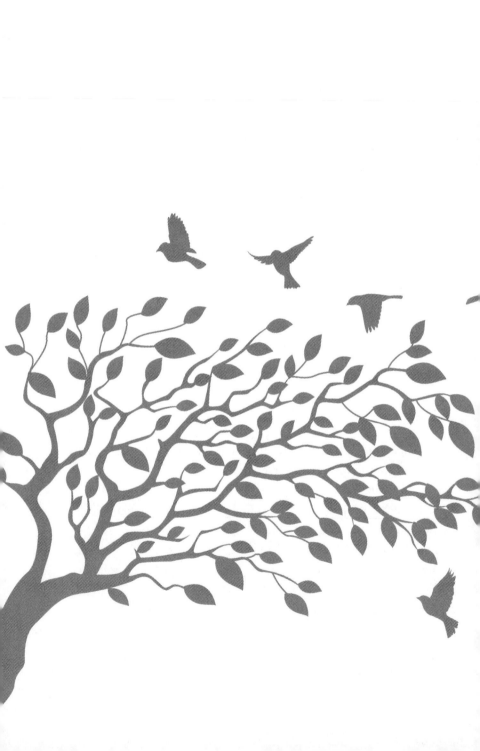

*The humanistic act of caring reveals
that we never outgrow our need for
love and understanding.*

Contents

Foreword

Some forty years ago I arrived in Canada from the United Kingdom. Under the good auspices of the Sisters of Charity of Montreal (the Grey Nuns), the Provincial Government of Manitoba, and the University of Manitoba, I was able to initiate the first palliative care unit in Canada at the St. Boniface Hospital in Winnipeg.

Mrs. Helen Allison was appointed head nurse for the new program. Her previous experience in social work and nursing was an attribute, and reminded me of my mentor in England, Dame Cicely Saunders. It soon became apparent to me that this resemblance was not merely superficial. Helen, like Dame Cicely, was highly intelligent and deeply committed to the field of palliative care. She was empathetic, perspicacious, mature, and competent. She was also an excellent teacher and motivator of those she supervised, and was dearly loved and respected by her patients and their families. To the medical staff, Helen was a highly valued and trusted colleague. It is very appropriate that she should now share her skill, knowledge, and insight with others.

Stay, Breathe with Me by Helen Allison is a brilliantly conceived addition to the existing literature on palliative care and caring. Helen's approach, through storytelling, is the most natural and appropriate method of teaching. It is a work that will undoubtedly be of great practical value and comfort to many patients, their families, and friends. Professional readers will certainly be able to identify many of their own patients in the vignettes that she presents. Likewise, I believe that this book may well encourage many more to seek a satisfying career in palliative care, and will extend the skills of those already working in this most important health care domain. Furthermore, it will be worthwhile reading for all health care practitioners, and not least for all physicians and priests! The lessons that we can learn from the dying are essential to all areas of our lives, professional and private.

For many years, as a specialist physician and a Catholic priest, I have taught that human beings can derive great benefits through suffering. Palliative care is, and always should remain, directed primarily towards the relief of the destructive and negative dimensions of pain and suffering, but we must never fail to maximize the very real opportunities presented for positive growth, maturation, and reconciliation. My own life has been especially influenced by the heroism of Pope John Paul II, and his Apostolic Letter, *On the Christian Meaning of Human Suffering* is, I believe, a masterpiece of spiritual discernment. As a teacher of Moral Theology I will now recommend that the Pope's great work should always be read in conjunction with this new masterpiece written by my dear friend Helen Allison.

—Dr. Rev. David Skelton MB, BS, DM, MRCS, MRCP, MRCGP, FACP, M DIV.

The Gift of
Compassionate Medicine

M atron, once a colonel of an army medical unit, demanded
exceptional care for hospitalized patients. Her standards
included cleanliness and order. In her presence one felt as if on
parade. Her command and words of wisdom: "Nurse, identify
yourself!" remain forever in my mind.

Revealing one's identity in communication with another
is surely an open invitation to our storytelling selves. But my
experience in a large teaching hospital as float nurse (replace-
ment for absent staff) denied me the opportunity to listen to
the patients' stories. Busy activity on borrowed time distanced
hospital staff from patients.

How could this be *care*?

Was the aim of treatment tied solely to skillful repair?

I began to think of illness as a drama. But without reading the patients' scripts, I was miscast, an uninformed extra, no
more, no less. I saw the patients as wounded heroes, who were
out of reach—their interesting lives on hold, their stories untold,
the passion of their souls excluded from their treatment notes.

And what of their fears?

As I walked through the hospital on my way to the Outpatient Department, I stopped to answer a patient's cry.

"Nurse! Nurse! Come quickly. Something terrible is hap-
pening. A lot of doctors have been called to Room 23."

Grasping my arm, her eyes wild with panic, she said, "Some poor bugger's had it!"

Distressed and anxious, this patient had conjured up an image that mirrored the fears of her own impending surgery. She was unaware that the hospital's code twenty-three signaled nothing other than a doctor's private telephone call and did not bode bad tidings.

Yet is it any wonder that patients are often filled with dread?

Hospitals are busy, foreign places, filled with mysterious codes and words, complex machines, and hurried staff. As a system, the hospital, just like a prison, is a closed system. You, the patient, are assigned a number, given a gown, and expected to obey orders. For the seriously ill and their families, the result is often one of great intimidation and feelings of distress.

Hospital caregivers are often more familiar with patients' blood counts and oxygen levels than patients' names. And often they forget that each patient has a doctor within, one that understands the unique manifestation of his or her discomfort and distress, one that knows when things are not right. Within this wisdom lies important information regarding the impact of pain and suffering—the unique characteristics of which are often revealed within their story. This wisdom of the patient is crucial because it contains pertinent information that is essential to enhance patient care.

———

We must never forget that serious illness is a drama of body, mind, and soul where symptoms and suffering cannot be separated from the person who is ill. Indeed, it is the wisdom of the patient that can guide the healer's hand. To alleviate suffering, we must embrace the human side of illness and view the patient, not as a set of symptoms, but as a hospitalized person and injured storyteller, with a unique understanding of the manifestation of his or her illness. Sadly though, in our modern, high-tech hospitals, the voices of the seriously ill are rarely heard and often silenced. And busy activity on borrowed time creates false barriers that distance medical staff from their patients.

This insight of the patient as an injured storyteller with healing wisdom to share was reinforced in my mind by a most unusual and unexpected event.

I was unprepared for the task at hand when I encountered a group of depressed outpatients. My assignment was to encourage their participation within a therapeutic group session. This seemed outlandish, because I knew nothing of the circumstances or sadness of their individual lives. And I lacked knowledge of mood-enhancing techniques. I felt myself on shifting sands and was forced to face my fear of failure.

I introduced myself to the silent group of seven patients, and then on a sudden, last-minute impulse, I offered them a workshop on "Sexuality and the Art of Care." As if wakened from some deep stupor, these seven unknown patients sprang alive, bright-eyed and alert. They had cast aside their gloom.

Given the opportunity to converse about sexuality and the art of care, their apathy fled the scene. And what was set in motion was an evocative, humorous narrative of life and living.

In this real-life drama, the participating patients led the way as protagonists, authors, and playwrights of their living scripts. Identities were revealed, tenderly reaching into childhood, connecting each of us with the cycle of events that had shaped our lives. Our unrevealing masks and self-imposed boundaries simply disappeared. I was richer for the knowledge that we shared.

The outcome of the workshop on "Sexuality and the Art of Care" was far-reaching and impactful. Through our community of sharing with open hearts and deep-listening ears to the lives, wounds, and worldviews of one another, the seven participating patients found an anecdote that raised their moods and bolstered their self-esteem. Miraculously, those patients discovered their doctor within, and that doctor set them free.

This experience with the group of seven patients taught me the humanitarian principles of compassionate care: that no one ever outgrows the need for love and understanding; that if we listen deeply to another person's story, if we reach towards them without judgment or opinion, we can enter that space of shared humanity and universal human needs, a space where suffering can be eased. It is these same humanitarian principles that lie at the heart of palliation and the art of care.

⸺

When caring relationships honor the unique aspects of our deepest selves, those relationships bring solace and comfort when sadness occupies our minds. No truer is this than when grief and loss cross our path, as inevitably they do throughout our lives. Yet ours is a society that attempts to hide these painful states, as if revealing our sorrow and our vulnerability is a shameful sign of weakness, rather than a natural expression of pain and heartbreak. To alleviate suffering, we must openly acknowledge and embrace all aspects of the human journey, including those of grief, illness, loss, and death.

I recall the time when as a student nurse, aged seventeen, I faced a reality that profoundly changed my life. A baby less than a year old, so perfect yet so critically ill, died while cradled in my arms. The head nurse intervened swiftly and with great skill. With compassion, she introduced me to the wisdom of the rituals that frame our lives. We gently bathed the precious infant child, swaddled him in fine, soft linen, then laid him to rest with a profusion of snowdrops placed upon his chest. This ritual honored the infant's death and acknowledged the presence and reality of our grief.

Although I did not know it then, that wise head nurse had introduced me to the philosophy of compassionate palliative care. At its core, palliation is the humanitarian act of caring, of reaching toward a wounded other, with a helping hand, a nonjudgmental mind, and an open, listening heart.

———

Our modern medical system excels at rehabilitation, acute care, and saving lives in situations of emergency. But its aggressive, scientific focus on symptoms, technology, and cure has blinded it to the person behind the illness. And, as a result, it has lost sight of the art of care. Today, medical knowledge is monumental. But sadly, the meaning of suffering has been obscured by the science of technology. This negation of suffering, especially in incurable illness, constitutes a major concern for all of humanity. Given that medicine is capable of extending life, surely medical practitioners are morally responsible to soothe the suffering of the seriously and chronically ill.

The relief of suffering ought to be a key principle of health care and a basic human right that applies to every person in need of compassionate care.

The time has come to revive the art of care. Palliation with its humanitarian principles of compassionate care can shine a guiding light. Palliative care teaches the importance of removing the false barriers that separate caregivers from the ill. It reveals the healing power of presence, of deep nonjudgmental listening, and of ongoing sensitive dialogue and communication, because it understands the healing, compassionate power of being heard and understood. And it embraces the wisdom of the patient, with respect and dignity, incorporating that wisdom into the management of their care. This living exchange of shared humanity allows the seriously ill to retain their unique sense of self and as much independence as possible, thus preventing the exacerbation of suffering that inevitably arises from an enforced state of helplessness and dependence.

The tender, nonintrusive nature of palliative care offers comfort to the seriously ill and their families. To palliate is to share and to care with humility and respect. When cure is no longer possible and life hangs in the balance, medical expertise in the management of pain combined with compassionate palliation provides a humanitarian approach that seeks to ease suffering at life's furthest shores.

To contemplate a serious illness is an awesome thing. Yet contemplation provides a source of meaning, and meaning can bring relief. And so, over the decades in hospitals and hospices and within family homes, I listened with an inquiring, feeling mind to the voices of my seriously ill patients:

"We're living, thinking persons. Can't you see?"

"Don't tiptoe 'round us. We're not dead."

"We need to share your laughter. And your tears."

"Scold us if you must. But please do not desert us."

"Don't try to protect us. Let us be who we are."

"We want to be full participants in the plan for our care."

"Don't judge us. Accept us."

In listening with an open heart to the patient's story of what it is like for him or her in the moment, we can begin to understand the reality and the nature of their suffering. This is what it means to "walk the patient's way."

The scene is now set for the drama to unfold as we embrace the human side of illness. My job as palliative nurse, medical social worker, storyteller, and mother of a critically ill daughter is to guide you through this narrative of illness and relief from unseen pain.

My one request of you, dear reader, is that throughout these pages, you read the term "patient," not as an identifier of a set of symptoms, but rather as a hospitalized person and, most importantly, an injured storyteller.

From the hearts and souls of the seriously ill and their families, here then are their stories.[1] They are the heroes who journey life's further shores. I honor their memory and acknowledge the gifts of wisdom they left behind. Let this wisdom guide us in our quest to embrace the healing art of care, to bring heart back into health care and compassion for those who need it most.

---

1. To protect the identity of patients, families, and caregivers, names and places have been changed.

"All I ask is to be heard and understood"

The Person Left Behind

He held up his hand as if to silence her. "No more questions!" But she persisted. It was her right to ask questions. She feared another stroke and needed to tell him of her terror. But the brain specialist had no time to listen to her story for he was doing medical rounds. So he turned his back and walked away. With dismay, she overheard her doctor say, "See what we have to put up with? Is it any wonder we need time away?"

Had he, this so-called brain specialist, no compassion? Had he no understanding of the person left behind? And she, a patient with a tumor on her brain, was shamed into silence and left alone with the terror of unanswered questions.

At times, silence serves only to magnify unspoken fears related to illness. A seriously ill person faces both an unwanted label and the challenge of being identified as a patient. This unenviable role sets out conditions and stipulations that are detrimental to the person who is ill. For example, the role of patient deprives a person of their independence. Patients are expected to conform and to obey their doctor's orders. And at times patients have no say in their plan of care. It is as though the patient is rendered mute and dependent. Surely this is contradictory to our understanding of the nature and relief of suffering.

Those who have challenged this impropriety are notable in their field of medicine and their names are recognized in the literature as advocates of compassionate palliative care. They include, among others, the late Dame Cicely Saunders, founder and former medical director of St. Christopher's Hospice in England; Dr. Balfour Mount, founding director of the Royal Victoria Hospital Palliative Care Services, Montreal; and Dr. Eric J. Cassell, clinical professor emeritus of health care policy and research, Weill Medical College, Cornell University, and author of many books and publications.

In terminal illness, physical pain is heightened by the mental anguish of multiple losses, including loss of independence, loss of body function, fear of isolation, and fear of death. Mental anguish, a constituent of suffering, must not be ignored. Dignity is paramount to the quality of patient care. No patient should ever be heard to say:

> "Yes, you named my pain. But unable to find a cure, you simply analyzed my symptoms and offered me nothing but cold logic."

> "How could you understand? You refused to listen when I told you of my suffering."

"Who will walk my way?"

A letter written by a friend reveals the reality and the impact of an unwanted illness and points to the many-sided aspects of pain and suffering. The writer of the letter was seriously ill. Her troubled thoughts spilled across the page: "I'm scared, but I will conquer fear."

What she asked for was the understanding of her friend. I heard her plea.

"It's not a storm that soon will pass away. It's more a loss of meaning in my life. I am weary and full of strange unease. The doctor was vague. He talked of positive tests with negative results and none of it made any sense to me. I told him of my pain. Pain that never goes away. But what he said made me shut my ears. Yet I heard him say cancer and palliative care. I'm to go to a hospice facility as soon as there's a bed. I've never heard of hospice or palliative care. I need you here! Come and stay. Help me find my way."

Her brave words, scrawled across the page, cried out for understanding, hope, and compassion. "No need for gloom. No need for clever answers to questions never asked. For where are answers to be found? Answers that explain life's ending? Others might respond with answers that are mere conjectures of their mind. What is to be done? Who will walk my way?"

Humanitarian Principles of Palliative Care

The relief of pain and suffering in critical illness
is a basic human right
that should apply to anyone in need of healing care.

The Management of Advanced Cancer Pain

When we are strangers to catastrophic illness and loss of self, we fail to understand pain's complex presence. Advanced intractable tumor pain is neither docile in nature, nor easily controlled, for it is both a physical and an emotional experience that dwells within the mind. The emotional aspects of never-ending pain have a social dimension that is tied to our self-identity and to the identity of our family.

When the doctor tells us that we are ill, we, in response, compose a story of what it means to be ill. Hoping to discount the information we have just received, we file our story deep within our mind. But when the dragons in our story, known by their frightful names of Fear, Pain, and Change, begin to rule our lives, we have lost our way. For in this odd new state we become strangers to ourselves.

Yet when you listen to my story about the person that I am,
your presence and awareness offers comfort and freedom
from fear and change.

In an ideal world, the standard of health care would be raised to the highest level. Hospice programs and palliative home care would be accessible to everyone in need of compassionate relief from suffering and pain. But we do not live in a perfect world. Nonetheless, advances in the science of medicine have made it possible to relieve pain and suffering in catastrophic illness.

In 1984, medical specialists in pain management developed a treatise entitled *Cancer Pain: A Monograph on the Management of Cancer Pain.*[1] The report, promoted by Health and Welfare Canada, provides knowledge about the treatment and relief of intractable pain in terminal illness. Information on the availability and effectiveness of analgesics and narcotics in pain control is provided in the *Monograph,* together with details of medication scheduling and the necessity of patient and family participation in pain assessments and developing treatment plans.

The *Monograph* is a valuable resource that challenges the false beliefs that pain in cancer is inevitable and untreatable. The *Monograph* also challenges the irrational belief that narcotics administered on a four-hourly or six-hourly pain regimen create a state of somnolence and drug addiction. On the contrary, a pain regimen that incorporates a treatment plan of care maintains the patient's comfort level and prevents the occurrence of breakthrough pain or pain that is out of control. An alert, comfortable patient, whose pain is contained within manageable limits, determines the effectiveness of the pain medication.

The wisdom contained within the *Monograph* provides a road map for health care clinicians in the provision of compassionate patient care. Moreover, what is presented in the *Monograph* is reflected in the experiences and the stories of patients and families described in this book.

Art and Science

> *I would rather know what sort of person has a disease than what sort of disease a person has.*[2]
> —Hippocrates

Medicine is both an art and a science, but there are times when the art of medicine is not practiced. The science of medicine requires systematic study in the pursuit of knowledge. Art, on the other hand, seeks to understand the essence of its subject. Thus science measures and observes the object of its inquiry, while art attempts to portray the characteristics and uniqueness of its subject. The combination of art and science is progressive in nature and embraces humanity with its person-centered approach in the provision of care. The patient's participation in the management of their illness is one of the primary goals of palliative care.

While analgesics reduce the intensity of unremitting pain, all too often the core of suffering remains. Yet it is the patient who holds the key to the knowledge that reveals the impact of pain upon their person. Pain is known and experienced by the person who suffers and endures it. And that knowledge is fundamental in forging the partnership of interpersonal patient care.

But how is pain perceived?

Pain may be defined in words that ultimately fail to capture and express the full meaning and dimension of suffering. On the other hand, the characteristics of pain can often be revealed within the story of the person who suffers. Stories are the conveyors of facts, of a reality that challenges, captures, and invites inquiring minds to venture into unknown places where suffering's awesome presence hides.

We are fellow travelers in the pursuit of healing care. But health care clinicians who do not listen to the patient's story, who negate the assessment of the patient's pain, must think again. Believing that you know what is best for a patient in unremitting pain reveals intolerable arrogance and ignorance. Everything must be done to alleviate a person's suffering, including consulting with the patient; anything else is inhumane.

In earlier times, the family played a crucial role in caring for the seriously ill. But the family of today is often small, headed by a single adult without benefit of grandparents or other relatives, and often lacks essential support in times of life crises. Moreover, in this age of transition, of an aging population and changing family structure, we tend to expect that others, including health care professionals, will care for our troubles and our dying.

Yet because of the multidimensional aspects of catastrophic illness, it is beyond the scope of any single individual, or any single discipline, to offer a comprehensive service that supports the needs of patients and their families.

Despite these challenges, great strides in the alleviation of suffering have been made.

Dr. Cecily Saunders provided scientific knowledge, understanding, and hope to patients and families in the provision of compassionate end-of-life care. She dedicated her life to the alleviation of the physical, social, and spiritual pain of patients and families under her care. The work of Dr. Saunders and St. Christopher's Hospice embody the humanitarian principles of palliative medicine and the pursuit of knowledge in the management and relief of unremitting pain.

Palliative caring is a combination of art and science in the pursuit of quality patient care, where collaboration between patient, family, and professional caregivers is required. In essence, a team approach is employed. The hospice team is multidisciplinary, drawing upon a diverse pool of knowledge and wisdom in an effort to resolve some of the complex problems that cause suffering.

The participation of patients, families, and significant others within the hospice team serves to enhance the quality of care for the terminally ill. Palliative care honors relationships of mutual trust and respect, as observed in the patient-doctor relationship. This relationship is a working partnership that invites communication and collaboration in assessing pain and determining a plan of care. When both patient and doctor work together in tandem, one behind the other, a partnership of trust is achieved and the dignity and self-worth of the patient is restored.

Historically, the development of hospice and the provision of palliative care were sponsored by charity and dedicated volunteers served as caregivers. Today, while charitable donations continue to support the high cost of providing this exceptional care, palliative care has become highly specialized in the management and relief of advanced tumor pain.

Unfortunately, the introduction of new procedures in relation to patient care challenges the status quo, and sometimes fosters opposition. A case in point was the opposition towards Dunira Hospice, described later in this book. That opposition was calmed only when the community itself rallied to defend and preserve Dunira's dignified, altruistic care for patients and families by establishing a hospice trust.[2]

Opposition to palliative care may also be related to the high cost of hospice services. But perhaps the greatest antagonists to palliative care come from our own fear of bleakness and loss of independence, our denial of human mortality, and our morbid fear of death.

To palliate is to comfort, support, understand, and relieve suffering. Palliative care and hospice care are synonymous, identical in usage and meaning. Palliative services extend beyond the familiar doctor-patient-nurse relationship, because the combination of medical knowledge, patient wisdom, and family relationships constitute total patient care. Patient and family participation within the hospice team counteracts despair and helplessness, and serves to restore hope.

The profound contribution of Dr. Saunders and St. Christopher's Hospice proved beyond a doubt the humanitarian benefits of palliative care. Surely that begets the question: *Is not the relief of pain and suffering a basic human right that should apply to every person in need of healing care?*

---

2. See the chapter, *Dunira Hospice: Rite of Passage.*

Children in Need of Palliative Care

Finding ways and means to build bridges
to those most vulnerable.

The altruistic nature of palliative care is medicine without boundaries or barriers. A hospice represents a dedicated community of health care professionals who provide healing care for both adults and children.

I recall a visit to a children's hospice in Paris, France, that gave validity to my research into the alleviation of suffering in terminal illness. Housed within a large teaching hospital, the children's oncology unit offered palliative care to seriously ill children. From outlying areas in France and other Latin countries came parents with children in need of invasive cancer procedures. They sought miracles and found shelter and care within the bosom of the hospice unit.

An open-door policy at the hospice provided options for small patients. Youngsters in remission from their illness stayed for short terms with a revolving-door approach that allowed them to come and go as required. Children no longer in remission had parents within reach, as mothers or fathers slept in hospital cots beside their children's bed. The hospice provided additional accommodations for family members close to the children's unit. And parents dressed in hospital green mingled with the staff as participants in the caring, communicating team.

One day at the children's hospice, I stopped to ponder what a young child, like little Monique, with no words to tell about her day might say. Maybe she would tell us something like this:

> *In this place that is a world apart,*
> *there are toys and hugs and silver stars,*
> *and Sesame Street as well.*
> *But when you're six years old,*
> *it's hard to tell the nurses how you really are.*
> *When there are no words, no words at all*
> *that tell about my pain, I show my nurse the*
> *little print that lives beside my bed.*
> *Five round faces paint a picture of what it's like today.*
> *And when I choose the fifth face that's crumpled up in pain,*
> *I get a gentle hug and something sweet*
> *that makes me want to sleep.*
> *Soon it will be story time*
> *with all the monsters gone.*
> *And before I go to sleep I will see the silver stars*
> *as they dance and drift away.*

To relieve the suffering of a sick and frightened child is to enter into their world and discover their poignant view of illness.

Caregivers who come with needles, medicine, and harsh treatments need to find a way to reach the troubled child.

It may well be a fleeting thing, but there are those who magically walk right through an invisible door and join the wondrous world of the child. They are the human magicians, who chase away fear and pain. These special people hold the key that opens a very special door. The key is to establish a connection with the child, one of trust.

Anatomical Puppets in the Art of Care

Many times it has been said that patient participation in the management of their illness counteracts fear and helplessness. But when you're a child, it's hard to tell the doctor how you are. Yet the wonder of the child's imaginative mind strives to find a way to tell about their day. Through symbolic gestures a child is able to communicate the experience of their reality to the adults in their life.

A poignant example of this was little Abby and her puppet. When Abby came to know her puppet, she found a make-believe guru who changed the circumstances of her life.

The remarkable story of this four-year-old child who was diagnosed with leukemia was televised in a newscast discussion that introduced Abby and her surrogate twin, a life-like puppet. Abby's puppet was her soul mate. She was Abby's second skin. Before the puppet entered her life, Abby suffered the trauma of intravenous drips, lumbar punctures, radiation, and chemotherapy, until a wise puppet maker from Manitoba brought comfort to a seriously ill child. And like the shaman of long ago, the creator of the puppet reached Abby's creative mind and did so with a look-alike puppet that bestowed meaning and a way to share a sick child's pain.

Velcro openings on the puppet's back revealed the spine where the doctor's needle went to get rid of the nasty cells that made Abby unwell. Velcro openings in the puppet's arms were the place where the medicine went to make Abby strong. And when the medicine did its good work, Abby and her puppet wore lace caps, because that helped their hair to grow.

Treatment modalities make no sense to a young, sick child. But Abby's understanding of her illness grew from her empathic understanding of her friend, the puppet. Abby's interaction with her puppet was purposeful and meaningful to her caregivers and to herself.

The creator of Abby's anatomical puppet is a Winnipeg artist of the theater. "Her craftsmanship can be found in clinics and hospitals across Canada, the United States, and more than fifteen countries including Belgium, Japan, Australia, and Bosnia."[3] Shawn Kettner, creator of the therapeutic, anatomical puppets, entered into the world of sick and traumatized children in order to empower them and to mitigate their suffering.

An example of the use of symbolic language is portrayed by the artist Norman Rockwell, whose paintings and illustrations were presented in, among other publications, *The Saturday Evening Post*.[4] A copy of this artist's oil painting, *Doctor and Doll*, hangs on the wall above my writing desk. For me, the genius of this artist reflects his humanity and understanding of the child's reality. The painting illustrates a child who, with trust and thoughtful deliberation, presents her doll to the doctor for medical examination. The child's doll is imbued with human qualities and personifies the child herself.

The Anguish of Childhood Awareness

An emergency admission to the children's hospital with toxic shock syndrome left my granddaughter critically ill. Unable to speak because of the breathing tube, she communicated with her eyes. I saw her fear and the tears that filled her eyes. Splinted arms held her intravenous tubes in place. But the immobility of the splints across both arms was more than a seven-year-old child could bear. It was such a small thing to bargain with the nurse, who listened to my request to remove the splints. The nurse complied on condition that I continued to hold my granddaughter's hands. This simple act of palliation brought comfort to a sick and frightened child, who was then able to gently fall asleep.

I will never forget the miracle of my granddaughter's survival. Her recovery was slow and constant, thanks to the compassionate, caring hospital staff. Her discharge from intensive care was a giant leap forward for she was finally able to breathe on her own. When offered fluids to drink, the thought of chicken soup tugged at her mind. So she politely placed her order with the nurse, who gently and firmly told her, "No!" Without a word, this disconsolate little girl hung her head in a gesture of defeat. But Grandma, quick to respond, bargained once more and asked the nurse to strain the solids from the chicken soup.

To my granddaughter this chicken soup-consommé brought utter delight. She turned to me, whispered in my ear, "Grandma, you know everything!" Thoughts of going home soon followed and restored my granddaughter's hopes.

Staying with a fearfully ill child to hold her hands and make sure she had a bowl of strained chicken soup were but a few simple ingredients of compassion in the provision of her care.

Extended Family Members at Dunira

Children who came to Dunira Hospice to visit a parent, grandparent, or other relative faced a bewildering adult world where serious illness brought unexpected and unwanted change. While children were never patients at Dunira Hospice, they formed part of Dunira's extended family. And for those children, Lucy was a source of comfort. She was a hospice volunteer who never flinched in driving out the malevolent rascal named Fear. Lucy never raised her voice or made demands on anyone. Her enormous appeal came from her engaging personality. Lucy, the wheaten terrier, resembled a gentle lamb. She invited smiling conversation from almost everyone and children adored her.

Each year the Cathcart School Choir came in from the cold and sang Christmas carols at Dunira. And each year, participating patients, better known as the Whispering Songsters, joined the children's choir. The festive Christmas season was celebrated in Dunira's family room.

The tragic death of one youngster from the Cathcart School Choir sent shock waves through Dunira and left a primary school in mourning. The death of a child is impossible to comprehend. And at Dunira, Stephen's death came to symbolize the tragedy of terminally ill children everywhere.

Myra Bluebond-Langner, social anthropologist, author of *The Private Worlds of Dying Children*, lays bare the harsh reality of seriously ill children. Her tender book identifies the awareness of terminally ill children. She reveals how cultural values 'anesthetize' us to the needs of children who are fatally ill. The children who participated in Bluebond-Langner's research "Faced death with a great deal of understanding about the world of the seriously ill, and their place in it."[5]

Critically ill children suffer overwhelming responsibility when they attempt to maintain a state of normalcy by the denial of their illness. "The requirements for maintaining mutual pretense place[s] tremendous burdens on those involved."[6]

For a while Stephen and his parents played that game.

A Child in Crisis

Sick children need to talk about their fears, real or imagined. And they need to know that their parents and other adults in their life are worthy of their trust. Trust is basic to our human needs. Trust begets security and security keeps children safe from harm.

Stephen was a pale, solitary, little boy of nine. He loved school and was the top boy in his class. His adoring parents were professionals who encouraged his love of books. His teacher knew him as a young scholar who was often lost in thought.

One day in an empty classroom, Stephen sat at his desk, small and frail and silently alone. Startled by the gentle pressure of the hand on his shoulder, Stephen heard his teacher's voice. It reached him from afar. He heard the words, "Stephen, it's time to go home." But he did not respond. His teacher asked, "Is it just that you want to stay and finish your schoolwork?"

Stephen did not reply. He simply covered his left eye with his left hand and looked up, puzzled by her intrusion.

"Stephen, are you playing a game of hide and seek with just one eye?"

Stephen's reply was slow in coming. "My eyes are funny. They make me scared. But I'm a big boy and I won't cry."

The school nurse confirmed Stephen's alarming symptoms

of double vision, loss of balance, and fatigue. The neurologist confirmed Stephen's brain stem tumor. And all those who knew the little boy were overcome with grief.

Thinking to protect their only child from the trauma of his illness, his grieving parents attempted to conceal the fact that he was ill.

In denial of such harsh reality, Stephen's mother told her son, "Your eyes feel strange because you hurt your head when Dad drove you home from school. Don't you remember? Dad got bumped from behind and slammed into the curb. That's when you hurt your head. Your eyes don't like that sort of thing. And now they need time to mend."

Despite his mother's explanation, Stephen was not reassured because his world had changed. The doctor's medicine did not help his eyes, and he was tired and scared. Everything at home appeared the same, yet everything was different. Silence replaced his parents' laughter. Silence was an unwanted presence that followed him around. At home the silence seemed so strange, so inauthentic. And Stephen wondered, *When will this silence end?*

To conceal the fact that one's child is seriously ill and attempt to maintain normal relations creates a barrier between child and parent. The very act of concealment is fraught with uncertainty and fear.

But where are the answers for the parents of a little boy who is slowly dying? Is there someone who can tell them how they should behave? Because in grief, meaning and logic are nowhere to be found. What occupied their distraught minds was untold suffering. And they remained ignorant of the impact of their negative behavior towards their son.

In ancient times, the shaman would have brought compassionate wisdom, as well as cloakroom hooks where those parents could hang their unspoken pain.

It was Stephen's teacher who originally uncovered his suffering when she patiently listened and heard him say, "My eyes are funny. They make me scared. But I'm a big boy and I won't cry."

The appalling nature of this youngster's pain was obvious, and school staff gave Stephen and his family their unconditional support. Compassion, after all, is a combination of kindness and simplicity.

To ease Stephen's suffering it was important to continue where possible with activities that were meaningful in his life. And this became an essential part of his treatment and his care. Welcoming the former top boy in the class to continue at school, even as a part-time student, allowed Stephen to achieve a sense of normalcy. In effect, Stephen's part-time school attendance displaced the chaos of his harsh reality.

Stephen's parents finally broke their silence and gently told their son that although he was seriously ill, they wouldn't send him away to stay at the hospital, instead they would care for him at home. And because his eyes had not yet healed, they gave him talking books. His made-to-measure wheelchair was meant to keep him safe from the unexpected onset of dizzy spells. Stephen's wheelchair, donated by an altruistic society that supports sick children, was his greatest gift for it gave him freedom of choice and movement.

With awareness, understanding, and compassion, Stephen's teacher worked to embrace Stephen and heal his hurts. She used storytelling and the creative art of play to feed the eager minds of Stephen and the other children in the class. Stories of adventures set the children free as they identified with heroes who walked their way. And together with the teacher, Stephen and his classmates created a gem of childhood dreams and imagination. What a celebration their pantomime evoked, full of imagery and hope. And for a time, Stephen found release in the mysteries of his teacher's storyland.

Children shared the stories of the heroes in their lives. And the majesty and magic of stories told and shared were the antidotes for childhood solitude and childhood fears.

In memory of Stephen, the children in his class created an artistic composition in the form of a collage. The principal elements of their memorial collage grew from their compassion, understanding, and collaboration with one another. Those same elements form the heart of the altruistic nature of palliative care.

Wisdom Shared: Dave's Story

*Take time to listen deeply,
to hear the thoughts that weep within the mind.
Take time to hear the person who is ill.*

Illness robs a person of life's meaning, the security of established social roles, and familiar patterns of behavior. As such, illness robs a person of their self-identity and their independence. To understand the person who is ill, you must stop and listen deeply. You must stop to hear the unspoken fears that speed their labored breath and the anguish of a cry that pleads: "Please. Stay, breathe with me."

In other words, to become a privileged partner in the relationship of healing care, you must listen deeply with an open heart to the stories from the patient's *Book of Life*.

Silence without Meaning

Weeks before his admission to a nursing home, Dave Farmer was visited at home by his doctor. Dr. Best examined the sixty-seven-year-old Mr. Farmer. The doctor poked and prodded the place where pain had taken permanent residence, and he listened to the vibrant sounds of his patient's chest. The solemnity of the doctor's visit and the physical examination did nothing to calm Dave Farmer's fears. Tension filled those moments for there was no social interaction, no communication or social discourse between the doctor and his patient.

Without revealing his medical findings to his patient, Dr. Best conferred with Hilda, Mr. Farmer's wife. In a hushed tone of voice the doctor directed her to administer the painkillers he prescribed for her husband. The atmosphere was clinical and sterile, and Dave Farmer's fears related to his loss of health turned into nightmares. Dave sometimes caught snatches of conversation between Hilda and the doctor, and he wondered why they excluded him from their discussions. Other unanswered questions followed in quick succession. In silence, Dave questioned his situation, *Is there no cure for this vile illness?*

Dr. Best's visits left Dave Farmer depleted as waves of predictable, nauseous pain swept over him. The doctor's medicine brought him no relief. Unable to rest, Dave kept track of his pain. He waited for the telltale signs of the approach of yet another wave of sickening pain. Hilda, once so reassuring, tiptoed around her husband, offering him food that she had painstakingly prepared, food that he could no longer eat. Her worried, anxious face revealed her grief and served to feed her husband's black despair.

Was there not one person who would sit with him and listen to his fears? Why was Hilda now silent? She never was before. Was she trying to protect him? But protect him from what? Oh what weight, what anguish, in avoiding a subject that both Dave and Hilda feared. But to name and face that fear was more than they could bear.

Seven months had passed since Dave and his son, Steve, first discussed the future of the farm. Steve knew that one day he would inherit his father's farm, but never did he think that illness would intervene. Not once did it occur to Steve that illness would force his father's hand before he had time to prepare for retirement. But time is swift and relentless. Seven months had passed and everything had changed. Pain and illness occupied Dave's mind. The future looked bleak. Steve's optimism failed to reassure his father. Steve's words echoed in his father's head. "Don't worry, Dad. Things'll be fine. I'll look after your Black Angus cattle. You can guide me."

Unable to hush the chatter of his mind, Dave acknowledged that seven months was a mere fraction of time in the life of any man, especially one who had never faced a serious illness in his life. Dave had not bothered with the usual medical checkups because Hilda had kept all mishaps from her husband's door. They were partners, he and Hilda. Dave bore responsibility for the upkeep of his prize herd of Black Angus cattle, while Hilda ran the house and tended the young animals in their care.

Farming and animal husbandry was the life that husband and wife had made for themselves, and Steve shared his parents' toil. Hilda's skill and master craft was her ability to manufacture small miracles on the farm. But no miracle was strong enough to make Dave's illness disappear.

With a feeling of foreboding, Dave knew that he had reached the crossroads of his life. His journey ended at an intersection. And at that intersection the road split off in different directions. Without a map to guide him on his way, Dave set forth, but the path that he had taken ended in a dead end, an undeniable blind alley.

Dave had lost his health. He had lost his way.

Institutional Care

Dave Farmer was admitted to Dr. Best's nursing home. Lack of sleep, anxiety, and pain muddled Dave's thinking and left him with no sense of time or place. Confined to a small white room with side rails on his bed, a room that signaled death's hidden presence, Dave asked, "Is this my prison?"

And in response, a nameless voice responded. "Mr. Farmer, you are a patient in Dr. Best's nursing home."

"How long have I been here?"

Once again the same crisp voice replied. "Eighteen hours by my time."

Who owned that voice? Distraught, Dave called out, "Hilda! Steve! Where are you?"

Confused and restless, Dave needed to flee from everything that clouded and befuddled his mind. Desperate to escape his confinement, he grasped the railings on his bed and shook them hard. But his actions went nowhere and robbed him of his strength.

Once again the faceless, nameless voice scolded him, hushed him as though he were a child, and ordered him, "Go to sleep!"

But sleep was the furthest thing from Dave's mind, for sleep enslaved him with fearful dreams of drowning pain.

Dave longed to talk with his only son. Steve would understand his father's plight. Steve would rescue him and remove him from this strange place. Yes, Steve was a beacon in his father's life, a beacon that would light this dark and empty place. "Hilda! Steve! Please come. Help me forget my pain."

In the presence of his family, Dave was centered, his point of reference and self-identity secure. But confined to the nursing home, Dave's identity had somehow disappeared.

What did it mean, this thing called "extended care"? To

focus his mind, Dave set himself a task. He pondered the words "extended care." Exactly what did they mean? Was it a trick to fill this place with helpless people? People who no longer questioned the meaninglessness of their reality? Dave thought that to claim the name "extended care" was a matter of hypocrisy and insincerity. So he renamed the place where he now lay captive, christening it "Dr. Best's Custodial Care."

Dr. Best and the nursing home staff ignored Dave's voice. They treated the farmer as if he were a child. He was allowed *no* say in the events or circumstances that surrounded his life. His voice was ignored. Dave felt abandoned. His appeal, urgent and pleading, fell on deaf ears. Not one "custodial caregiver" listened or responded when he cried out, "Take me outside and shoot me. My pain is pure hell."

Communication Breakdown and Paternalism

Hilda heard her husband's cry, but she didn't know what to do with an abrupt and surly doctor and an insensitive health care system. So with a sense of urgency and outrage, Hilda developed her own plan of care for Dave. But how could Hilda's plan succeed with a doctor who was distant and a system that was custodial and inhumane? Dedicated to easing her husband's suffering, Hilda persisted. She understood that hope and compassion are essential to the care of the terminally ill. Even in good health, all of us need hope, because without hope, we may shrivel up and die.

Hilda resolved to change the impact of the outmoded ideas that were being imposed on patients in the "extended care" facility. Hilda's plan of care for Dave included two nurses qualified in palliative care. Hilda engaged the nurses to provide dignified comfort care for her husband. Both nurses listened to the fears that heightened and prolonged Dave's pain. And once again, Dave knew the joy of being heard and understood. Hilda informed Dr. Best that she had hired two private nurses to care for her husband. And in turn, the nurses proposed a meeting with Dr. Best, in order to assess his patient's pain and implement a plan of care.

But reality, cruel and unyielding, revealed that palliative care was foreign to the institute Dave Farmer had christened "Dr. Best's Custodial Care." Tension filled the air and muttered rumblings reached the ears of Dave's hired nurses: "Just who do those palliative nurses think they are requesting a medical review by Dr. Best?" "Don't they know Dr. Best will reject any care plan they come up with?" "How dare they try to change the rules! Who do they think they are?"

Dave's hired nurses upheld the belief that those who opposed palliative care would eventually concede and come to realize that suffering is the enemy, a wrong that must be righted. Surely, their common goal was to improve the quality of the patient's care. Why then did Dr. Best and his custodial staff distance themselves from a dying Dave Farmer? Were they without compassion? Were they unable to see a dying patient as a living person in great distress, a person who sought and who needed understanding?

Dave's nurses were committed to ease their patient's suffering and to this end they enlisted the support of the clinical pharmacist on Dr. Best's staff. The pharmacist was the one member of the nursing home who supported palliative care. She was an advocate for the alleviation of Mr. Farmer's unremitting pain. Together the nurses and clinical pharmacist combined efforts to reveal the intensity of Dave's endless pain.

Dave's palliative nurses introduced Dave to a medical tool for pain assessment—in this case, the *Knoll Pharmaceutical Pain Scale*. With the use of this tool, Dave identified those areas of his body where pain took its toll. The able farmer confirmed the duration of his pain and stated that lack of sleep influenced his moods. The palliative nurses carefully recorded this all-important information on Dave's body chart.

Pain assessment tools provide a simple way for patients to describe and measure their pain. For example, a pain scale may resemble a small rule measure calibrated in numbers from zero to five, plus the combination of five colors. Zero on the scale indicates no pain experienced and is correlated with the color blue. While the number five is correlated with the color red and signifies that the patient is experiencing extreme pain. Palliative caregivers use pain scales with hospice patients to assess their level of pain prior to the implementation of a pain regimen. (Sensitivity, though, is required for patients from other cultures, who may understand the meaning of color in a way that is different from our own. For example, the color red in western cultures signifies, among other things, intensity and danger, while in some eastern cultures, the color red is associated with luck, long life, and happiness.)

Pain assessment tools are proven medical instruments employed in the management of chronic, persistent, and malignant pain. When the palliative nurses listened and carefully recorded Dave Farmer's pain, the integrity of his subjective pain experience was acknowledged. Dave told his caregivers that his pain was "drilling, burning, killing, nightmarish." Dave Farmer's documented pain record provided the palliative nurses with a visual image of the intensity of his pain and revealed its unpredictable behavior.

The Negation of Suffering

The documentation of Dave Farmer's pain should have been recognized as a valuable medical instrument, showing the need for the administration of narcotics to relieve his advanced tumor pain. But Mr. Farmer's detailed pain assessment was unacceptable to Dr. Best, who refused to change his prescribed medical orders.

Dr. Best discounted the validity of his patient's experience of pain. He rejected the pain assessment and dismissed its value and accuracy. Without further consultation with Mr. Farmer or his family, Dr. Best made his intentions known to nursing home staff. He flexed his medical muscles and proclaimed to those within hearing distance, "Mr. Farmer is under *my* care and *I* will tell *you* about his pain." With those words Dr. Best may have retained control over his patient, but he discounted any compassion or humility.

Dr. Best may have felt empowered by the belief that he alone understood the suffering of his patient. But it was a grave error in his thinking. One must ask: How exactly did Dr. Best acquire this knowledge of Mr. Farmer's suffering? The mystery was profound since Dr. Best, through lack of time, did not map the course of Mr. Farmer's pain. In fact, Dr. Best discounted Mr. Farmer's pain assessment and ignored the expertise of the clinical pharmacist, whose knowledge of the principles of narcotic use in chronic cancer pain was extensive.

Dr. Best questioned the motives of the clinical pharmacist as an advocate of palliation. She was a member of the nursing home staff, but she had crossed the line through her consultation with Mr. Farmer's private palliative nurses. Dr. Best also discredited the palliative nurses with the words, "How dare they question my authority. They are not employees of this nursing home. They are nothing but the hired handmaidens of Mrs. Hilda Farmer."

Was Dr. Best aware that, in assuming the "Lone Ranger" approach to patient care, he had ridden roughshod over the feelings of Mr. Farmer and his family? Dave Farmer had placed his trust in Dr. Best. But by assuming power over his patient, Dr. Best had betrayed Dave Farmer's trust. And since Dr. Best lacked the ability to understand Dave's suffering, the austere doctor may have clung to his power but was rendered impotent in offering any help at all. Further, by discounting his patient's experience of pain, Dr. Best denied Dave Farmer the right to participate in the management of his own care.

Any health care professional who negates a patient's communication and participation in relation to their illness is paternalistic. Paternalism is symbolic of the imbalance in power between the omnipotent parent and the helpless child. In health care, paternalistic behavior creates an ethical dilemma, where the rights and responsibility of both patients and caregivers are diminished. A patient's rights bring into question the decision-making process and the necessity of mutual consent for treatment that affects prognosis and outcome.

The most important part of all communication is to listen—to hear and understand what is being said. But this takes time. It takes time to stop, to open one's mind, and to listen deeply in an attempt to grasp the meaning of what is being said. There is no doubt that when a doctor does not take the time to stop and listen to a patient, but instead proceeds on the basis that he or she knows best, the art of medicine is lost.

Hilda Farmer raged against her husband's doctor for the harm done. She questioned his promise of "extended care" and condemned the system that granted him license to practice medicine.

Nor could Hilda Farmer erase the thought that lingered in her mind. *No farming man would ever stand aside and allow an animal to suffer such unremitting pain.*

Dave Farmer's son, Steve, regarded Dr. Best as a braggart—remove his doctor's power and what was left?

Dr. Best had been unmasked; he had no knowledge of palliative medicine, no knowledge of the detailed wisdom written in the *Monograph on the Management of Cancer Pain.* Perhaps that wisdom was something only other doctors could understand.

Instead of wisdom, Dr. Best revealed his need to retain control when he proclaimed, "*I'll* tell *you* about my patient's pain."

Why did Dr. Best allow such foolish words to linger in the air? Knowing what is best for a seriously ill patient in unremitting pain is a contradiction in thinking, because common sense tells us that it is the patient who experiences pain. It is the patient, and perhaps the patient's family, who understand the impact of pain and the suffering that follows in pain's wake.

When the physician discounts the severity of a patient's pain, the patient's suffering is increased because there is no doctor-patient relationship, no working partnership. And therefore no meaningful exchange of information can take place. The physician who negates pain as an individual, subjective experience has rendered the interdependent relationship between doctor, patient, and family null and void. In consequence, the intrinsic value of the patient as a person and a participating partner-in-care is denied. And the patient suffers.

Dave Farmer told his nurses, "I'm not afraid to die. Death will bring relief. My doctor sees me as a diseased body. He's written me off. But now I have the measure of the man. He's a friend to no one. Not even to himself. My illness is of no consequence to him. I expected something better. I thought he would have some answers for my pain. But how can he know what I am going through when he doesn't even look my way? I wanted to tell him what it's like to be ill. But he doesn't want to listen. So why am I here? I need to be at home."

The *Monograph on the Management of Cancer Pain* clearly states that:

> "Pain is always subjective. Pain is what the patient
> says it is and not what others think it ought to be."[7]

Dave's nurses were responsible for the provision of compassionate palliative care, but the environment of Dr. Best's nursing home proved detrimental to their patient. In reviewing the conditions that surrounded Mr. Farmer, his nurses identified the elements that exacerbated his suffering and were morally reprehensible. The conditions imposed on Mr. Farmer that hindered the provision of humanistic patient care included:

- Medical mismanagement of advanced cancer pain

- Negation of the patient's suffering

- Negation of the patient's wisdom

- Paternalism

- Custodial climate of hostility

- Opposition to palliative care

- Loss of patient dignity and hope

By identifying the conditions that increased his suffering, the nurses heard and incorporated Dave Farmer's wisdom into an alternative plan of care. Dave told his nurses, "I need to be at home." And in hearing him, his nurses presented a contingency plan for patient and family care.

The nurses requested that Hilda take her husband home.

"Yes," Hilda replied. "I will take Dave home. But how will we manage?"

Dave's nurses reassured her. "We'll continue to provide hands-on care for Dave at home. And we will contact Dr. Andy, who is committed to palliative care. We work with Dr. Andy throughout the community. He's a family doctor with several palliative care patients of his own. You'll like him. He's just like the old-fashioned family doctor of long ago whose very presence improves your health. And Hilda, when Dr. Andy comes to the farm, invite him for tea. He'll love your home-baked buttered scones."

Dave Farmer spent the last few weeks of his life at home. And during that time he was relatively free of pain, thanks to Dr. Andy. Surrounded by the events that shaped his life, his son's stories of their Black Angus cattle, and the presence of friendly neighbors, Dave regained the freedom to be himself. With dignity and comfort, Dave Farmer concluded his life in the security of his beloved farm home.

Paul's Journey

Often invisible to the naked eye,
suffering is distress that is magnified by the mind.

To understand the origin of advanced cancer pain requires a combination of skill, ongoing assessment, and review of noxious symptoms. But to identify pain's origin is not in itself enough, since the meaning of illness is modified by the mind. Spiritual beliefs, culture, economic circumstances, family values, personal aspirations and limitations—all play a major part in how we experience pain and how we relate to illness. Age is also an important variable that influences pain and suffering. Invisible to the naked eye, suffering is distress that is magnified by the mind.

The findings of my own research with seriously ill patients revealed that youthful patients may not accept their terminal diagnosis. Awareness of death's approach heightens the value of life—a life of fulfillment denied the young who are gravely ill. Without doubt the manifestation of pain in catastrophic illness must be viewed in the context of the patient's age and life experiences.

The alleviation of suffering in terminal illness is complex and demands a partnership of care and trust. Trust grows in an atmosphere of compassion, active listening, commitment, and cooperation between patients and their caregivers. Understanding the words that each person shares is an essential component in the alleviation of advanced cancer pain and suffering. To lose sight of the patient as a person and participating partner in the caring relationship is contrary to palliative care.

Paul was twenty-eight years old when he was diagnosed with a spinal cord tumor. Paul's loss of health must be viewed in relation to his personal history, his aspirations, his hopes, and his dreams. To review Paul's medical prognosis with the object of making his noxious symptoms the focus of treatment would be to lose sight of Paul the person and deny his humanity.

At the tender age of ten, Paul inherited a large old mountain bike from his uncle, Bob. Undaunted by the height of the bicycle saddle, Paul rode his new bike standing on its pedals. And standing on the pedals he dreamed his dreams of becoming a powerful athlete and racing cyclist. Bicycles carried Paul into manhood; they were his passion. He rode them, repaired them, and sold them. And for a time, Paul basked in the glory of his achievements in cycling.

Paul's wife Linda was his greatest fan. Paul and Linda dreamed of a future full of joy as they awaited the birth of their first child. But just as dreams are conjectures of the mind when the body is at rest, in waking the veil of sleep is lifted from our eyes and reality confronts us. Awake we sometimes see our dreams as mysterious illusions.

The birth of their baby daughter brought Paul not one ounce of joy, because sickness had taken hold of him and happiness had fled the scene. Paul found himself pursued by an invisible assailant, an assailant that robbed him of his energy. Tired and irritable, unable to respond to his newborn child, Paul withdrew and locked himself inside his house of pain. Linda saw that her husband was a shadow of his former self, more phantom than person, and she didn't understand why she could not reach him. The old familiar ways of doing and being were gone. The signposts had fallen down. Paul had lost his way. Who, or what, was the unseen presence that caused him to despair? Rooted in his illness and his pain, preoccupied with the injustice of his life, Paul lost sight of his wife and baby daughter. Paul's unseen assailant robbed the strength from his once powerful legs, and there were times when Paul could not feel the ground beneath his feet.

Following a collapse, Paul was admitted to a local hospital. There, a stoic Paul received the information of a tumor growing in his spine. But Paul refused to accept his doctor's diagnosis. He convinced himself that the tumor was not, ". . . a growing thing. It was a lifeless obstacle to be overcome."

Obstinate and determined, Paul resolved to defeat the obstacle that blocked his way. Had he not throughout his life overcome all obstacles that stood in his path? Slowly, Paul formulated a plan of action. And the more he thought about the plan, the greater his hopes grew. As for the cost of his plan? It didn't matter. All that mattered was the removal of the "obstacle" that robbed him of his health.

Let no one block the way or calculate the cost of a cure, for Paul was on a mission and his mission was unassailable. Blinded by unreal expectations and clinging to his hopes, Paul discounted all caution in his search to find a cure.

Yet how could Paul or Linda heed the voice that cried, "Beware"?

They were vulnerable and scared and they faced a truth that was impossible for them to bear.

So Paul and Linda searched for Utopia and fled to a place where "miracles" were common. They escaped to Never Never Land, where mystery and fabricated miracles seduced, deluded, and raised false hopes. And so it was in southern climes, Paul and Linda sought and found a superior "God," a miracle worker who offered Paul a cure. But sadly, Paul's superior "God" was a charlatan who offered fraudulent claims of miracles through the power of healing hands. These so-called healing hands made no use of scalpels; instead they promised to melt all tumors and make them disappear. And while these so-called healing hands falsely offered a cure, they ultimately left Paul and Linda penniless and poor.

Disabled by adversity, they returned once again to Canada. Paul visited his family doctor, who gently talked to him of the reality of his situation. There was no cure. Only then did a reluctant Paul accept an admission to Dunira Hospice.

But Paul was a reluctant patient. His self-imposed silence and avoidance of the palliative caregivers was not in keeping with his need for total patient care. Every day Paul nursed his grief and held it up to view. During his waking moments his mind festered on his problems. And in silence, his anger mounted until, in a rush of explosive rage, Paul's barriers finally tumbled down.

Who Will Understand?

When Jean, the hospice social worker, knocked at Paul's door she unknowingly entered into his rage. In a fury Paul threw his urinal straight at her. The urinal struck Jean directly. For a moment she froze with shock. Then in lightning speed she reached Paul's bed.

Jean's instincts told her to quell Paul's rage. But how?

The answer came through the healing power of touch. With purpose and determination, Jean clasped Paul in a tight embrace. And this she did to contain her own anger as well as Paul's explosive rage. Jean held him tight as one might hold a youngster to quell the force of destructive rage. Still holding Paul she scolded him, as a mother might scold an angry child. Loudly Jean exclaimed, "How dare you strike me with your urinal!"

But this was not the moment to talk to Paul about his responsibilities as a patient. As matters stood, Paul regarded his caregivers with contempt. In his mind, they had robbed him of his dignity and his life.

Paul raised his voice and wept. "I don't want to be here. I've got no future here. But I can't go home. I was an athlete. But not now. Not anymore. I was a husband. But not now. Not anymore. I'm no longer a man. But you're a woman. You wouldn't understand. I'm not even a father to my baby girl. Christ! I'm twenty-eight years old with a tumor that's left me half a man. Can't you see? I'm paralyzed below the waist."

Paul stumbled through the fury of his words. "You dare talk to me as if you know me. But lady! You don't know who I am. Once I fought to win races. But win or lose, there was always honor at the end of the race. That's where the glory was. Racing to the end like a hero. But this is another race. There's no glory here. There's no honor. There's nothing but darkness."

And Paul wept for the bleakness of the journey that lay ahead.

Paul's Discovery

Two members of the palliative team believed that in recounting the highlights of Paul's young life something remained to be salvaged, something that could bring him a small measure of hope. Dr. Daniel brought his person-centered skills to Paul. The wise doctor did not focus on the miracle of cure, nor on the loss of dreams. Instead, doctor and patient shared their ideas of goals that were within Paul's reach. And in listening, Dr. Daniel offered Paul support, thus empowering a despairing young man.

Judy, the occupational therapist, was the other person who entered Paul and Linda's life. She offered them encouragement and presented them with challenges. Judy encouraged Linda to learn the new skill of transferring her husband single-handedly from his bed to his wheelchair. And Judy challenged Paul to accept a day pass home, and when comfortable, to extend the pass and spend a weekend home. Paul and Linda met the challenges that Judy sent their way. And those challenges became the acts of courage that gave meaning to their lives.

Judy became Paul's pathfinder. As the occupational therapist at Dunira Hospice, Paul discovered Judy in the craft workshop. The familiar smell of leather in Judy's workshop filled Paul's senses and reminded him of bicycle saddles and races to be won. Judy's large, imposing person placed Paul at ease. She was full of life, and her laughter reached the place where Paul's good feelings had daily drained away. With the lightest touch, Judy plugged that leak for good. Judy was not indifferent to Paul's suffering. Indeed she offered hope as she chased his misery away with her dark Australian humor. But never once did Judy enter into Paul's "ain't it awful" scene.

The simple task of creating leather crafts in a place where Judy ruled the roost gave Paul a sense of direction and a reason for being. Paul invested himself in the hobby of creating small leather goods. The pliable leather responded to his touch as he worked to mold and change its shape. And as he worked, Paul discovered that he had taken strides to change his point of view about his situation.

Was it Judy's colorful stories that brought about this change? Or was it her Australian pictures and postcards that covered the walls of the workshop that led Paul to venture in his mind to places unknown?

The reason for the change in Paul's feelings about himself didn't matter. What mattered was that Paul had accepted that he was now a person with a different point of view. There were choices to be made and choices brought him hope.

Then came a turning point in Paul's metamorphosis and a major step forward into life. This turning point was instigated by his daughter, Fiona, a mere infant child. Paul's new vision shone from his own wee lass. But how did Fiona accomplish this remarkable feat? Fiona, pure and innocent of intent or purpose, simply opened her chubby arms to Paul and with a dimpled smile uttered the sound, "Dada." Two syllables, yet the music of that precious sound pierced her father's loving heart.

The final word on Paul's journey came from Dr. Daniel, who said, "Paul is not yet out of the woods. But he is making progress. Along the way he will confront detours and blind alleys. Be that as it may. But it's important for us to remember that Paul has reinvested himself in his family. He's getting on with what is important in his life. Can anyone ask for more?"

Dunira Hospice: Rite of Passage

*Perhaps the greatest obstacle to palliative care
is to deny that life is finite.*

The story of Dunira is one that must be told. Dunira is a hospice in its early-middle years and to me, a cornerstone of palliative care in Canada. Yet at its inception, Dunira's location, within an acute care hospital, resulted in controversy.

To ease the burden of the sick, Dr. Daniel, a humanitarian and specialist in palliative medicine, invested himself in the creation of Dunira Hospice. But early in Dunira's ministrations to the critically ill, rumors of euthanasia reached Dr. Daniel and alarmed the hospice staff.

Those who fostered the belief that palliative care was just another name for euthanasia sent shock waves through Dunira. Without a doubt, ignorance is the source of false beliefs, of blame, and of fear. To equate palliative care with euthanasia is an error in thinking that serves only to foster paranoia. As such, those who sought to discredit Dunira and palliative care attempted to force the closure of the hospice.

At the time of these events, Canadian law regarded euthanasia as a criminal act. Doctors who ended a person's life through the administration of a lethal injection had, in the eyes of the law, committed a crime punishable through prosecution.[3] In effect, the rumors of euthanasia at Dunira cast blame on Dr. Daniel for a crime he had not committed.

Despite the passion of Dr. Daniel's words, they fell on unhearing ears. "Euthanasia is a human tragedy," he said, "for it is suffering unleashed and unattended. Euthanasia represents our failure to alleviate suffering." With the wisdom of the sage, Dr. Daniel stood firm, constant to his patients and their families, for he believed that the humanitarian principles of palliative care would be upheld.

Dunira's mandate of care had been discredited. Yet everyone could see that Dunira's mandate was beyond reproach, since patients, families, and the community at large benefited from the hospice's palliative care and caring. And yet within the acute care hospital, Dunira's staff was frequently questioned: "What is palliative care?"

By definition palliation is non-invasive, tender care that offers comfort and support to patients and their families. Care of the terminally ill identifies the importance of meaningful dialogue and participatory relationships. To palliate is to share and to care with humility and respect. When a cure is beyond humanity's reach, medical expertise in the management of pain combined with compassionate palliation preserves the patient's dignity. Palliative care seeks to alleviate suffering in serious illness.

What folly to equate euthanasia with palliative care! What folly to accuse Dr. Daniel of the practice of euthanasia! What wrath would fall upon the heads of those who sought to close Dunira Hospice! For in this small Canadian town, the com-

3. For more information on this subject, see the section, *Euthanasia and Physician-Assisted Dying.*

munity held sway. The community rose up and confronted the Board of Hospital Directors with factual information. And with tenacity, the community peeled away the covers of deception, laying bare the true nature of palliative care. Notable towns-people defended and honored their investment in Dunira by establishing a hospice trust that ensured Dunira a safe rite of passage. The fault-finding condemnations of the unenlightened crumbled to dust.

A united community had saved its hospice.

Palliative care is progressive and multidisciplinary in nature. The humanistic nature of palliation dissolves professional boundaries, inviting open communication between professional disciplines in an exchange of knowledge for the benefit of all. At its heart, palliative care offers the hope that compassionate care will continue and ensure dignity and respect at life's conclusion.

Yet despite all that has been written about the humanistic quality of palliative care, questions remain:

> *Is the master craft of understanding still beyond our reach?*
> *Is suffering in illness misunderstood and "inaccessible"*
> *or is it simply beyond our capability?*

My daughter knew the story of Dunira. She understood the meaning of palliative care. Palliation was her life support while she remained at home. But later, her confinement in the health center of an acute-care hospital changed her point of view. With great dismay, I heard my daughter's words. "Nobody here knows about palliative care. It's all just pretend." Was this her illness speaking? I read the thought that lingered in her mind: *I want to die at home.*

My daughter's troubled thoughts were a symptom of her illness. A symptom that expressed the suffering of her body, her heart, and her mind. When everything hurts and life holds no meaning, suffering is interminable.

As a basic human right, palliative care should be available to all critically ill persons. Palliative care represents a community of caring relations. Above all, palliative care seeks to reach the person behind the illness and attempts to ease the patient's fearsome burden.

Nowadays, palliative care, or hospice, is sometimes located within the confines of a hospital, stands alone in a separate building, or is offered at home. I recall my meeting in Paris with a specialist in palliative care. We talked about the greater need for palliative caring within patients' homes. And we concluded that when family members are unable to care for their loved ones at home, other options should be provided.

The story of Dunira[4] continues throughout the pages of this book. Dunira Hospice provided a meeting place for courageous men and women who journeyed there and imparted a powerful message:

Death is not the enemy to be feared.
The enemy to be disarmed is
the lack of humility and the lack of understanding
of grief, illness, fear, and pain.

---

4. Throughout this book, "Dunira" represents an amalgam of palliative care services.

Palliative Care Services Reviewed

To connect at the junction
that separates the living from the dying
requires compassion, commitment, and understanding.

The purpose of conducting a review is to acquire factual information concerning the nature and outcome of the subject in question. At Dunira, team meetings provided the information required by the palliative care audit, which identified both the limitations and the positive aspects of palliative patient care. Dr. Daniel, or his delegate, chaired the weekly multidisciplinary team meetings. Invited guests included medical specialists who provided knowledge on the management of intractable pain. The assessment of hospice patients included a review of pain, symptoms, and level of patient comfort. Problems were identified and their resolution sought.

The complex nature of pain management and care for the terminally ill is mirrored by the diversity of the hospice team. This diverse pool of knowledge is focused on the relief of pain and suffering. Hospice team members are committed to the creation of an interpersonal community of care. Patients, family, doctors, nurses, pharmacists, social workers, clergy, physical and occupational therapists, and hospice volunteers comprise the hospice team. At Dunira, patients and family members did not attend the formal weekly team meetings.

Nursing reports, created upon the arrival of all new patients, contained medical histories and were continuously updated throughout the day and night. These nursing reports provided ongoing communication and continuity for patient care.

At Dunira, less formal patient and family care meetings were arranged to develop pain protocols and patient care plans. Participating patients, family, and those team members best qualified to meet the patient's needs attended those meetings.

In addition to team meetings, and patient and family care meetings, Dr. Daniel reviewed patient deaths biweekly. The positive aspects of this review were considerable. Not only did the review identify those family members in need of support and bereavement counseling, it also offered support to caregiving staff who mourned their patient's death. Review questions included the following:

- Was the patient conscious or unconscious?

- Was the patient comfortable or in distress?

- Were families or friends able to express their grief or share their feelings with staff?

- Were family members given the opportunity to remain with the deceased in order to say good-bye?

- Was clergy notified of the death and present at the death?

- How is the staff feeling about this patient's death?

In addition, team members discussed the quality of patient and family care during the dying process. Dr. Daniel asked those in attendance:

- "What was done for the patient and family during the dying process? How were they supported?"

- "Did we as caregivers miss anything?"

- "What might we have done for this patient and family?"

- "What might we do for patients and families in the future?"

- "What have we learned from this review?"

Information gathered from the review was summarized and became a part of the patient's palliative care record.

Before we join a team meeting[5] as an invited guest, let's review some of the recorded notes of Marty, the night nurse.

Marty had never forgotten the rare gift of insight she had received from a beloved patient at Dunira. Marty's patient was an artist, a musician who played with a symphony orchestra. His illness had robbed him of his voice, leaving him unable to speak of his needs and fears. Marty bore witness to his anguish. Her caring presence reassured him, and a relationship of reciprocal trust was born.

---

5. The team meeting is described in the section, *The Hospice Team Searches for Answers.*

Thinking to comfort Mr. Musician, Marty said, "I have brought you a collection of Brahms's cello sonatas. Perhaps the sounds and the vibrations of the music will bring you comfort." As the musician listened to the sonatas, his body relaxed. Marty witnessed the knots of fear disappear. Music was a powerful opiate that worked to ease his pain.

Mrs. Lambie, Person Unknown

Nurse Marty needed no persuading about the soothing effect of music on the mind. With the insight she had gained from Mr. Musician, she understood that music is a medium that safely cradles and soothes the child within. And if music cradles and soothes the frightened child, could music stem Mrs. Lambie's fear? Could music ease Mrs. Lambie's spiritual pain?

Marty's notes revealed that Mrs. Lambie had been admitted to Dunira at 0600 hours. She was accompanied by her husband Sam, and was received into care moaning and wailing in a high-pitched voice.

Concerned for his wife's state of distress, Sam had told Marty, "Norma is deeply religious. She was brought up on the teachings of the Bible. But God has not answered Norma's prayers. She's angry. And she's turned her back on her church and her faith."

Marty was aware of the unspoken fears of patients in crisis, when illness occupies their mind. Sensitive to the language and sounds made by her patients, Marty believed that Mrs. Lambie's lamentations were an expression of her spiritual pain. The apostle Paul gave meaning to spiritual pain. We moan because we desire new life and wholeness. We wail in a high-pitched cry to lament the circumstances that have befallen us. Mrs. Lambie was angry with her God. Her world was upside down. Death stared her in the face. Where would she find peace? What was to be done?

In compassion, nurse Marty asked Sam, "Would the gentle music of a lullaby bring comfort to your wife?"

"Norma likes hymns," Sam answered with an audible sigh. "But she won't thank you for any music right now. Her mind is fully occupied in the belief that God has abandoned her. Nothing else is important, nothing else matters."

Determined to relieve his wife of her burden of suffering, Sam tried in vain to meet her needs. While he had no knowledge of what brought relief to his wife, he understood her unspoken words, her every look and gesture. And without direction, Mrs. Lambie held her husband responsible for her comfort and her care.

Nurse Marty provided a thumbnail sketch of the behavior of Mrs. Lambie's pain. Mrs. Lambie had been a patient at Dunira for a mere four days, less than a fraction of a moment in the life of any person. To her palliative caregivers, Mrs. Lambie was a stranger. No one knew her story because she had kept her canvas blank. Yet her care was about to be reviewed by Dunira's hospice team gathered round the conference room table.

The Hospice Team Searches for Answers

Let's stop a moment and observe the hospice team in action as they search for answers to the seemingly insurmountable problems related to the provision of patient care. In listening, we may hear what sounds like a family argument when voices are raised in defense of questions asked and answers given.

Dr. Daniel reminded the team that Mrs. Lambie had been a patient at Dunira for less than a week. Then he asked, "What have we accomplished in the provision of care for Mrs. Lambie?"

His question was met with silence, yet he continued, "Thinking to preserve the dignity of Mrs. Lambie and out of consideration for her roommate, we moved her into a private room. But in moving her we've increased her isolation. It is obvious to me that we do not understand this patient's reality."

Dr. Daniel paused for a moment, then asked, "Why has Mrs. Lambie cut us off? Did we bring on the difficulties that we presently face? Should we have done things differently? Does anyone know why we've failed to meet this patient's needs? How do we feel about the void of silence that prevents us from reaching Mrs. Lambie and her husband, Sam?"

Head Nurse Claire told the team, "Mrs. Lambie's husband was ill at ease when he brought his wife to us. And Sam's still distressed. He was his wife's main source of support at home. When he asked me if he could continue to provide her personal care, of course I agreed. But it's obvious to me that Mrs. Lambie hates being here."

Sister Beatrice offered no comments, which was unusual, since she made a point of meeting all new patients on the day of their admission. Most patients enjoyed Sister's visits, and she always greeted them with a welcoming smile. Her Irish stories were a warm invitation that helped the patients relax and sometimes invited their laughter.

Dr. Daniel turned his attention to Sister Beatrice, but

before he could question her she said, "Now don't go looking at me. I've no answers for you."

Not to be dissuaded from his task, Dr. Daniel persisted. "Come now, Beatrice. I'm sure you can shed a little light."

"No, I can't. I can't shed any light at all because Mrs. Lambie refuses to speak to me. I'm a Catholic nun, and she dislikes Catholics. God bless her soul! So that's just it. Mrs. Lambie holds each and every one of us at arm's length. How can there be any meeting of minds when there's no communication?"

"Oh, this is sad. Where is the dignity in any of this?" asked Dr. Daniel.

The social worker added, "I think we must accept our own imperfections and gracefully bow out. Perhaps resignation is all we have. It may well be that we've failed to bridge the gap with Mrs. Lambie because we need help. After all we can't fix everything by ourselves. Maybe Mrs. Lambie cut us off because she is terrified of death. And for the first time in her life she understands that life is temporary."

In hearing the discussion between members of Dunira's team, are we to conclude that the opinions of the caregivers led them to make value judgments? And if so, is the team guilty of defensive behavior that serves no purpose other than to isolate them from their patient? In reviewing the care of Mrs. Lambie and the discomfort of Dunira's team, the big picture has not yet been revealed. Indeed, we may be looking in the wrong direction.

Marty, the night nurse, drew our attention to the behavior of Mrs. Lambie's pain and the tyranny of suffering that she expressed with her continuous moaning and high-pitched wailing. Marty's notes also revealed the impact on other patients and families who shared Mrs. Lambie's space.

Team members concluded that a breakdown in communication was the culprit that separated Mrs. Lambie from her caregivers. While a breakdown in communication is a serious matter and a detriment to patient care, other matters needed consideration.

Dr. Daniel identified a lack of dignity for both Mrs. Lambie and her husband. The social worker argued that the team needed help because, as she said, "We can't fix everything by ourselves." Some situations lie beyond the capacity of palliative care, however well-intentioned. The team acknowledged that there was no meeting of minds. And Sister Beatrice expressed her hurt feelings.

But no one pointed to the fact that during her short stay in hospice, Mrs. Lambie had refused to participate in the management of her care, hence the expectations for a patient-caregiver relationship had not been realized. Moreover, Mrs. Lambie's strange, discordant sounds had caregivers dancing out of step. Is it possible that difficulties arose because palliative objectives for patient care had somehow been changed? And if the goals of patient care were changed, who made the change?

Mrs. Lambie absolved herself of all responsibility as a patient in care. She bent and broke the rules through her non-participation with her palliative caregivers.

Palliation represents an *interdependent* partnership of trust between patient, family, and caregivers. This caring relationship is one of doing *with* the patient, not just *for* the patient, which nurtures their sense of independence and dignity. But a belief that patients must accept the philosophy of palliative care would be to deny them freedom of choice.

Mrs. Lambie did not wish to be a patient at Dunira. But

concern for her husband's well-being had led her doctor to admit Mrs. Lambie to our hospice. Her admission to Dunira represented a loss of control and was perceived by Mrs. Lambie as an unwelcome intrusion in her life. Was Mrs. Lambie's continuous wailing a protest against her unmet needs? Was her self-imposed withdrawal a manifestation of suffering beyond endurance? During her short stay at Dunira not one member of the caring team had come to know her story or understand her needs.

Mrs. Lambie taught her unwelcome caregivers to keep their distance. She was enabled by her husband, who willingly submitted to each of her demands. Mrs. Lambie refused to communicate or participate with the palliative staff. Consequently, there was no plan for nursing care. Sam was the vehicle through which she met her needs. Sam enabled her to vent her rage at God and humankind. Sam, loyal and reliable, was held captive by his wife. And blinded by compassion, he accepted the daunting task of providing her with nonjudgmental care.

But what of Sam and the suffering he endured? Sam was everywhere, but nowhere within sight. Many questions remained unanswered. Was Sam the sacrificial lamb, a loyal and morally responsible victim caught in a trap of honorable intentions?

And was Mrs. Lambie a person who saw no need to accommodate others, no need to hide her dislike for her palliative caregivers? Was self-loathing a manifestation of her persona?

Most importantly, is a fatally ill person deserving of whatever brings them relief, no matter the shape or form? And if so, can hospice caregivers accommodate antisocial behavior without blame?

These are difficult questions and perhaps there are no answers.

Nevertheless, the role of palliative caregivers is to bridge the gap that separates the living from the dying. And to connect at that junction requires compassion, commitment, and understanding.

"An Ancient Longhouse"

⟡

Dunira's family room offered a place of quiet retreat for patients and their families. Not by design did this oblong room take its shape or earn its disposition. Hospice families had fashioned it, making it a home away from home. Sofas and big reclining chairs stood in comfortable disarray around the unpretentious room, while brightly colored cushions donated by family members created a feeling of warmth. An old oak table sat squarely in the center of the kitchen, where someone would brew the morning coffee or make a pot of tea.

And on this day of major significance, one that belonged to Gordon and Grace, a wedding would take place. That such an event would be celebrated in the hospice family room was not at all unusual, since celebrations were commonplace. Birthdays and memorials were respectfully honored as part of living life within the palliative care community at Dunira Hospice.

The kitchen formed the heart and soul of Dunira's family room. And the kitchen was the place where Brian accidentally announced his presence in a most spectacular way.

Brian, a teen on the cusp of manhood, was tired and hungry, weighed down with concerns for his seriously ill grandfather. Preoccupied, operating as if on automatic pilot, Brian placed two breakfast eggs in the microwave. He had no knowledge of the workings of microwaves, no knowledge of their potential as an explosive device. An unsuspecting Brian simply placed his breakfast eggs whole and intact inside. How was he to know that he should have pierced the shells of the eggs with a pin?

Seconds later an explosion burst from the microwave. The remnants of the shattered eggs and shells descended like snowflakes that covered the entire surface of the old oak table. Stunned by the explosion and shocked by the mess he had made, Brian collapsed into one of the big reclining chairs.

Caring Comradeship and Harmony

Maria's voice reached Brian's tired ears. Maria was like the loving matriarch of Dunira's extended family. She said, "Now don't you fret. In no time at all, we'll clear away this mess."

The sound of Maria's voice transported Brian to a time of childhood. As Maria stood before him, he saw instead his mother's image and a sudden flood of long-forgotten memories came rushing to his mind. Oh, the magic in the memory of his mother's voice, her words like music to his tired ears, words of a distant time that danced across his mind in the stories he had once so loved to hear. And in those memories, Brian once again knew the pleasure of the smells and tastes from his mother's oven, the pleasure of warm cinnamon cookies, just newly baked. But that was so long ago. Why now was he remembering that time? And why now did he suddenly remember that at the tender age of seven his mother had gone to heaven? How he missed her.

Now, just nineteen years old and a student of anthropology, Brian was soon to face another major loss. His beloved grandfather was seriously ill.

Maria waited at his side. How could she know that in his grief Brian was not equipped with the logic of a peaceful mind? Brian longed to hide himself away, but Maria encouraged him to face the task at hand. She might have been the loving mother who coaxed her erring son. Nurtured by Maria's wise and gentle presence, Brian acknowledged his grief and accepted Maria's gift of friendship.

Brian viewed the world through the eyes of a social anthropologist. His interests lay in the study of the customs, beliefs, and social organization of mankind. For Brian, Dunira's family room represented "an ancient longhouse." He believed that the families who occupied the longhouse were a clan, similar to an extended family that cared for one another. Brian's concept of the longhouse gave purpose and meaning to his stay in the shabby, oblong room at Dunira, where every day family members faced the crisis of life's termination.

Not that Brian was simply an observer of the characteristics, customs, and habits of those who occupied the longhouse. He too had taken comfort from the nonjudgmental care of those around him, recognizing that both he and they shared a fearful vulnerability. Yet in spite of this vulnerability, each played their part in the caring palliative team.

To anyone who would listen, Brian was heard to say that since coming to Dunira: "I've learned a lot about living and I've learned about love without strings. My grandfather is very ill. And I've learned that it's okay to cry. I used to be afraid of death. But I don't feel that way anymore. When I finish school, I'll come back to Dunira and be a hospice volunteer."

Brian had gained an understanding of the resilience, humanity, and courage of the families in his longhouse. Brian's surrogate family was united in a bond of mutual respect, and through the comradeship of people in crisis, they had formed a self-help group unique in all its functions. More than once, Brian acknowledged the support that resided within the extended family at Dunira.

One day, Maria interrupted Brian's reverie when she arrived carrying small bunches of snowdrops, crocuses, and white heather. She carefully placed the late-winter blooms on the oak table in the family room. Brian noticed that Maria's chubby face was bright red from the bite of the cool wind that blew outside. Dark-blue shadows under Maria's eyes told him of the long hours spent at Dunira. Maria's husband was one of four patients in the large room at the end of the hall. Each day Maria made small Italian meals for her husband. And not once did she forget to tempt the palate of her husband's roommates with a delicacy from her kitchen.

Brian would always remember his first meeting with Maria, when his critically ill grandfather was admitted to Dunira. At that time, Brian's state of mind was one of worry and dread. Maria became his greatest ally, and he would always cherish the support she gave him. In the weeks that followed, Brian came to think of Maria as the compassionate matriarch of his newfound family. And he thought of Dr. Daniel as the wise sage who coached his hospice team in the art of caring for the patients.

Brian helped Maria arrange the flowers in vases. As Brian mused about the comfort and support he felt in the family room at Dunira, his thoughts were suddenly interrupted by a voice that had been held in check for much too long.

It was Sam's voice, the voice of Mr. Sam Lambie, a voice no longer in control. He was in a high state of excitability and was giving vent to his feelings. Sam behaved as if he were drunk.

But Sam wasn't drunk. He was overwrought and desperately needed to be heard and understood.

Sam clung to Brian's arm as if to steady himself. For the last five days at Dunira he had tended to his sick wife's every need. Mrs. Lambie had kept her husband always on the run. With the tenacity of one in sober self-denial and with no time for rest, Sam had slept on his feet as he soldiered on. Now spent, not a scrap of energy left and no ability to think straight, Sam pointed to the two paper bags that lay at his feet and said, "That's all. That's all that's left of her! She died this morning just before dawn. I can't believe she's gone."

Brian placed his free hand on Sam's shoulder and said, "I'm sorry."

"Don't be, I'm not," Sam said. "It was those guys down at the church. It was their prayers that kept her going so long. I asked them to stop praying for her. But they didn't understand that it was her time to go." Sam sucked in his breath, paused for a moment.

"Norma and me were married eighteen years." Sam wrung his hands. "Yet I never really knew her. The trouble was I never went to church. I'm not a church-going person. We didn't get married in the church. But surely a person doesn't have to go to church to be a good person? Norma thought I was a heathen. She tried to change my ways. In her eyes, I never measured up. I never amounted to anything. She never forgave me for not being a Christian like herself. I always wanted kids. But we never had any."

Sam paused to catch his breath. "Now that she's gone I can please myself. I'll be an uncle-at-large for all the kids that don't have a dad. And I'll be a volunteer driver for cancer patients."

Brian patted Sam's shoulder. "You're a saint, Sam. You gave and gave. And never asked anything for yourself. Don't reproach yourself. And don't forget us, Sam. We won't forget you. Come back and join the support group. Every Wednesday we meet and talk about important things. All the things that must be said. And we try to help one another find ways to make things better."

Both men fell silent.

Then they heard Maria say, "Sam, you will join us for coffee? It's newly brewed. And you need to know that the wind has a fierce bite this morning. So before you put a foot outside that door, get this inside you." As Maria said this, she placed before Sam a breakfast of bacon, eggs, and buttered toast.

Sam thanked Maria for her kindness, and she replied, "I think that you and me are in need of a hug." Then without hesitation Maria embraced him.

After the meal, Sam collected his two brown paper bags and offered a quiet good-bye. His departure left behind the memory of a sad, bewildered gentleman.

As we took our leave of Sam, we hoped that one day down some distant road he would cast away his victim self and add a new and different chapter to his *Book of Life*.

A Wedding at Dunira

Maria covered the old oak table with a cloth of crisp white linen and placed her bowl of late-winter blooms at the table's center. Other family members joined Maria to prepare the family room for an event that marked the day as one of great significance.

A celebration of the highest order was about to take place, a celebration that honored the union of Grace and Gordon in marriage. Gordon, gravely ill yet in full consciousness, pledged his love to Grace with the knowledge that his final good-bye would bring his bride a painful void. Sadness had taken its toll on the loving union of Grace and Gordon. Yet can any one of us avoid the weight of sadness and sorrow when bereavement separates us from the ones we love?

To those in despair, Dr. Viktor E. Frankl, author of *Man's Search for Meaning,* offers solace, understanding, and wisdom with his words:

> "Whenever one is confronted with an inescapable, unavoidable situation, whenever one has to face a fate which cannot be changed, e.g., an incurable disease, such as an inoperable cancer; just then one is given a last chance to actualize the highest value, to fulfill the deepest meaning, the meaning of suffering. For what matters above all is the attitude we take toward suffering, the attitude in which we take our suffering upon ourselves."[8]

And so it was we gathered round Gordon's bedside. His dying wish was to be wed. Grace, the reverend, two witnesses, and I stood in silence to honor the profound and meaningful act of marriage and to acknowledge this solemn declaration and affirmation of life. Gordon rallied for a moment and what we heard was the muffled sound of thunder as he lifted his voice, "Yes, I'm still alive." And he held up his face to be kissed.

Gordon, now that you are wed can you allow your mind to rest? And Grace, just newly wed, can you see that we are standing here for you? For we in hospice share both pain and joy as we walk the way with you.

The depth of our compassion was revealed in the ritual of the wedding celebration. And with unconditional love for the newlywed couple, Dunira's hospice families provided a simple wedding feast.

"Why does the night nurse wake me for my medicine?"

Ongoing dialogue and open communication
between patients and caregivers
defines the hopes of both parties and builds relationships of trust.

Angie was one of the first patients to be admitted to Dunira. Her gynecologist was responsible for her transfer from the main hospital to palliative care. Angie's loss of health was rapid in its progression.

Angie's pain was of such magnitude that many times her husband Tom heard her say, "Just let me die. Just let my heart stop beating."

Vexed and despairing, Tom accompanied his thirty-three-year-old wife to Dunira. The palliative team of Dr. Daniel, Head Nurse Claire, and Clinical Pharmacist Linda met with Tom and offered him support. They encouraged his participation within the palliative team. And Tom's contributions were to be major and significant in the management of his wife's pain.

Angie's Pain Assessment

Angie had been at Dunira for two short days when she told Tom, "My pain is getting better. But I don't understand. Why does the night nurse wake me for my medicine?"

Tom smiled at his wife and said, "Angie, what would you say to the kids in your class if they told you they didn't understand? Wouldn't you tell them to ask?"

Tom and Angie were teachers. They had no children of their own. But their pupils kept them in touch with the world of youngsters.

Angie soon discovered that the routine of morning care helped her to relax. Her primary bedside nurse was an able communicator and she painted pictures for Angie of life outside of Dunira. Conversation between Angie and her nurse was effortless and full of meaning. At times, Angie wished her morning care would last twice as long. She enjoyed the peaceful, unhurried camaraderie and the comfort of the soft warmed blanket that the nurse placed on top of the freshly made bed.

At Tom's suggestion, Angie asked, "Why does the night nurse wake me for my medicine?"

Angie's nurse sat down beside the bed. "Were you able to get back to sleep after being wakened?"

Angie nodded and waited for her nurse to continue. "Angie, your night nurse is your guardian angel. She wakes you because you need that medicine. The medicine has to go on working all through the night. While you sleep the medicine continues to ease your pain. But I'll bet you didn't know that the pain medicine has a life of its own. It loses its strength in four to six hours. And then it stops working. So if the night nurse didn't wake you, you'd wake up with heavy pain. That's why, without you having to ask, you get your medicine every four hours, round the clock, day and night."

Angie asked her nurse, "And is that why we trace pain on my body chart?"

"Yes, exactly. What you tell us about your pain and how it makes you feel is very important. That's why Dr. Daniel stops to study your body chart during his morning visit. That chart shows all the places where your pain lurks and hides. And when Dr. Daniel sits beside your bed and asks you to tell him what it's like for you today, what you tell him guides his management of your care."

She smiled and continued. "And as well as all of that, Angie, your nurse gathers up the facts about what makes you feel so ill. You might think your nurse is simply playing detective. But it's not some sort of game. We need to know if you're alert, or sleepy, maybe confused, perhaps a little dopey. All those facts are recorded as symptoms on your pain assessment record. And that's important because it's your pain assessment record that helps Dr. Daniel and the clinical pharmacist work out the medicines that will relieve your pain. Other symptoms, like loss of appetite, nausea, vomiting, and bowel evacuation, are also noted and are included in your plan of care."

"And by the way, Angie," the nurse added, "we depend on your husband. He tells us when you are sad, or scared, or angry. Those questions may seem like a drag. But the answers you and Tom give provide the hospice team with information that is important for your care. Without all those questions and answers we would all be in deep trouble. Trying to treat an illness without mapping the course of events makes no sense. Can you imagine treating blood pressure without measuring its up-and-down behavior? So, Angie, that's why we search for answers that tell us what we need to know about your precious self. Does that make sense? Have I answered your questions?"

"Yes. Now I understand why the night nurses wakes me for my medicine. And now I understand the different parts that come together to help manage my pain. Thank you, nurse. It makes sense to me now."

EMOTIONAL PAIN

It is not uncommon for seriously ill patients to lapse into despair when hope is beyond their grasp. A patient's expression of despair is a symptom of their emotional pain or suffering of the mind. The primary nurse is often the person who discovers the cause of a patient's distress.

During Angie's morning bed bath, Angie's nurse asked, "Can you tell me what's bothering you this morning?"

Angie turned her tearful face toward the nurse and said, "I want to drown this scary voice inside my head. It keeps saying I won't get well. What purpose is there in my life? All my life I've tried to please others. What a waste of time! Then there's Tom. Have I pleased Tom?"

Angie's failure to provide Tom with a child was engraved upon her mind. But to Angie, to leave a child without a mother was unthinkable. She knew firsthand the suffering of a child grieving the loss of a mother. At an early age Angie herself had been orphaned.

"I was twelve years old when tuberculosis killed my mother. I never got over her death. You never get over the loss of your mother! Grandma never talked to me about mother's illness.

She never talked about mother's death. Grandma's silence scared me. I was just a kid, but I couldn't help wondering if I had somehow caused my mother's death."

During morning care Angie talked about her childhood. She told the nurse, "Once there was a woman in my father's life. She tried to take my mother's place. Her name was Peggy. She was small and fat. In our house she played the piano. And she sang songs to my father. I hated her! When she sang I held my hands over my ears and wished she'd stop. One day she tied my mother's apron round her thick waist. I couldn't stand it. So I pulled away the apron strings. Then I hid my face inside mother's beautiful apron. And I cried and cried. I think my bad behavior sent Peggy away because she stopped coming to the house. I was glad. But my father was angry and sad."

By sharing her fears and her sorrows, a weight seemed to lift from Angie. And perhaps because there is nothing more precious than being heard and understood, the pain in Angie's pelvis decreased.

A delighted Angie was no longer able to trace the pathway of pain on her body chart. She asked, "Does this mean I'm getting better?"

Patient Rights

The meaningful back-and-forth dialogue with her nurses brought comfort to Angie. But it didn't last because suddenly Angie was thrust into the bleakness of a monologue that excluded her.

The gynecologist who had originally referred Angie to palliative care dropped in for an unexpected visit. His visit was formal as he assumed authority over his former patient. What he proposed terrified Angie. He told her that he hoped to use her as a "medical model" to advance his students' knowledge of obstetrics. Angie said nothing. She was too terrified, too intimidated and confused to know how to respond. Her silence led the gynecologist to believe that she had agreed to his proposal.

The gynecologist made no attempt to dialogue with Angie. His visit was a monologue and nothing more. But he took her silence as consent to participate in clinical teaching rounds.

This was an unethical and inappropriate request because the gynecologist had no medical jurisdiction over Angie. Blinded by an aggressive scientific focus, the gynecologist failed to see Angie as a vulnerable, desperately ill young woman in need of comfort care. Instead of Angie the person, the gynecologist saw only the manifestation of anomalous symptoms and the possibility to further his research. But Angie was no longer his patient; Angie was now in the service of Dr. Daniel, Medical Director of Palliative Care. Further, given the need for dignity and comfort care, it is unlikely that a patient in palliative care would consent to intrusive clinical examination by medical students.

Angie was seriously ill and her rights were being threatened. As a patient, Angie's rights allowed her to refuse participation in research and teaching procedures. But up until the visit by the gynecologist, Angie had had no need to consider or defend her patient rights.

Angie struggled between the need to please her gynecologist and her loathing of an examination by medical students. If she agreed with the gynecologist, not only would her own needs go unmet, she feared it would prove her weakness as a person.

The turmoil of this conflict brought Angie to the brink. Finally, she blurted out to her nurse, "I don't want this! I don't! But I'm too afraid to tell him."

"What is it that you don't want, Angie? Has someone made you angry?"

"It's my gynecologist. He'll ask me questions I don't want to answer. He'll examine me in places where it hurts. There's no dignity in this. Why do I have to have that horrible examination? And with all those students. I'm going to tell Tom to take me home."

Angie's nurse slipped into the chair beside the bed. "Angie," she said, "you don't have to take part in any teaching procedures. You have the right to refuse. It's your right as a patient." She went on to explain the principles and rights of patients:

> "The decision to receive treatment or refuse treatment is made by the patient, not by the doctor, whose role is to recommend and give advice."[9]

With obvious relief, Angie asked, "You mean I can say no?"

"Yes, Angie," the palliative nurse replied. "You can say no. And that'll be the end of it. It's your right as a patient to say no."

Angie took a big breath and let it out in a sigh. "Oh. I didn't realize." She paused before she continued. "But some weeks before I came to Dunira," she told the nurse, "I did sign a consent to participate in teaching rounds. Nothing happened. So . . . so I think I have to do it now anyway. I don't think I have a choice." Her words sounded heavy with resignation.

The nurse squeezed Angie's hand. "Angie, listen," she said, "the consent you gave prior to your admission to Dunira is no longer valid. The hospice team and Dr. Daniel are responsible for your care now. Dr. Daniel is your doctor now. And palliative care does not support invasive medical procedures in the name of research. That's contrary to palliative principles."

She patted Angie's hand to reassure her. "Listen, Angie, if you feel alarmed by an invasion of your privacy and you no longer feel safe here at Dunira, if you want to go home, we can arrange it. You can go home and the palliative care nurses in the community will keep an eye on you. They will monitor and assess your pain, just as we do here. They will teach your husband about your pain medicine."

With the nurse's reassurance, Angie visibly relaxed. Back and forth the women dialogued as Angie mulled her options, freely voicing her thoughts and concerns. And as she did, the tone of her words lightened as if the weight of worry and dread and false obligation had been lifted.

"If you choose to go home, Angie, there will always be room for you to return to Dunira," the nurse said. "But if you just want to go home on a weekend pass that can also be arranged. You have choices. But before any of your choices can be realized, Dr. Daniel will meet with you and Tom. The head nurse and the social worker will also be at that meeting to plan the details of your home care. Knowing that you have choices leaves room for hope. What are you thinking now? Has our conversation helped clear your mind?"

"Yes, it has," Angie replied. "I must talk with Tom. We have a lot to sort out. I like the idea of a weekend pass. So will Tom." And for the first time that morning, Angie managed a smile.

When Angie's former gynecologist proposed that Angie participate at teaching rounds it was morally and ethically irresponsible. Angie was critically ill and under the care of the palliative team. Her former consent had become both outdated and invalid. And it was fully within her rights as a patient to refuse.

Patients expect professional caregivers to be ethically and morally responsible. By the same token, caregivers have similar expectations. Just as patients in care expect to be treated with dignity and respect, their caregivers share a similar expectation. Ongoing dialogue and open communication between patients and caregivers reveals the hopes of both parties and builds trust in the patient-caregiver relationship. In palliative care there is no room for a one-way-only monologue.

PROTECTING ANGIE

Afternoons at Dunira were usually quiet, but the unfinished business between Angie's former gynecologist and hospice staff was soon to dispel all peaceful harmony on the unit.

A sudden commotion and angry words spilled from the nursing station down the hallway. The noise caught Claire, the head nurse, by surprise and she glanced up to spot an agitated hospital porter with an empty stretcher on wheels arguing loudly with Angie's primary nurse. Never before had Claire witnessed such a loud and unusual confrontation in the hospice. She rushed to the nursing station and demanded to know the reason for the commotion that had shattered the late-afternoon tranquility.

Angie's nurse was red in the face and clearly flustered. In a voice full of outrage, she blurted out, "What nerve! That gynecology prof still thinks Angie is his 'medical model.' But his department was told she had canceled her consent for his research. Angie's not going up there to be examined by medical students just so they can advance their learning."

With her usual calm, Claire told the hospital porter that a mistake had been made and that he had no authority to take Angie upstairs. Furthermore, no authorization would be forthcoming. Then, with purpose and quiet composure, she opened the door to allow the porter to remove both himself and his stretcher.

Claire considered the possibility that the senior gynecologist, a medical professor, might at any moment make an angry appearance on the unit. After all, she, a mere head nurse, had called into question his authority. With that in mind, she lifted the phone to inform Dr. Daniel of the incident.

Angie's nurse chimed in, "That poor porter's gonna get it in the neck when he returns with an empty stretcher and no Angie."

"No doubt he'll be told off," Claire replied. "But the problem is not his. The problem lies with the gynecologist."

It was clear that the argumentative porter had no knowledge of palliative care. He was simply following instructions. And, when prevented from doing his job, he had overreacted in an angry outburst.

Claire reminded the other nurses. "Angie is now under Dr. Daniel's care. She is seriously ill and requires gentle care, not some fact-finding investigation and exploration."

The gynecologist, blinded by scientific interest in Angie's anomalous symptoms, was simply pursuing clinical objectives of his own. His goals for research and development had, without doubt, obscured his view of Angie the person.

As the palliative nurses discussed the situation, Claire told them, "This is an unusual incidence. Not likely to be repeated. The only logical explanation is a breakdown in communication.

I've never seen anything like this in palliative care. Angie is dreadfully ill. And it's our job to protect her."

Claire then thanked Angie's nurse for her responsible advocacy and defense of her patient.

By defending patient rights, palliative care embraces the ancient art of healing. Those humanistic principles are embedded, honored, and protected by the very nature of palliative care.

Angie did not need to fear the recurrence of an unwanted intrusion or loss of personal dignity. Angie's palliative caregivers would protect her.

Jock, Brian, and the Sea Captain

*The healing power of camaraderie
and memories shared . . .*

Quiet, peaceful afternoons at Dunira ensured the head nurse precious time to visit with patients and families. Claire's visit with the retired sea captain found him propped up in bed enjoying a conversation with Brian, his grandson, and Jock, his roommate. The stately old gentleman was always at his best in his grandson's company. It was as if he marshaled his life's forces and energy to stay on course.

For Jock, the Scotsman, sharing a room with the sea captain was a recent event. But it was more than mere coincidence that the captain and Jock came to share their space.

Before his admission to Dunira, Jock had worried himself sick with fears about retirement. He was fifty-four years old, never married, and had no family. Work meant everything to Jock; the idea of retirement terrified him because he feared being alone with nothing to fill his days, nothing to anchor him in life. Then something more frightening than retirement forced Jock to give up his beloved work. Jock had terminal cancer. When the oncologist referred him to palliative care, Jock agreed without hesitation. Dunira offered him a safe haven, peace of mind, and the companionship of others.

The Joy of Camaraderie

Dunira's hospice team thought of Jock as a rough diamond and eternal optimist, who filled the empty spaces of his surroundings with vital energy. He was a man of heart and passion, and many found pleasure in his company. Jock was a storyteller supreme. And for those who listened to his tall tales, time quickly disappeared.

Jock's earlier fall from grace had no lasting consequence. He had reclaimed his dignity and was no longer on probation after the madcap escapade during his stay in the private room at Dunira, now occupied by Angie. It may have been boredom that enticed Jock to act without thinking. Whatever the reason, he caused himself a lot of trouble when he locked himself in the bathroom of his private room to consume a half bottle of whiskey. None of the nurses could arouse the drunken Jock from behind the locked door. Finally, security had to be called to release the unconscious Jock from his bathroom prison. Much to Jock's surprise, he woke to discover that he was now sharing a room with Brian's grandfather, the sea captain.

In no time at all, a reformed Jock found joy in doing small tasks for the seriously ill sea captain. The three men, Jock, the Captain, and Brian, formed a bond of friendship that surpassed all else.

Transfer to a semiprivate room was the best thing that could have happened to Jock, whose claim to fame was his work on the ferries of the west coast of Canada. The captain welcomed Jock's assistance. And Jock was happy to assume the rank of first mate. Indeed, Jock became the old man's right-hand mate. And with every passing day, Jock's dignity and independence grew.

Jock told his nurse, "I know it sounds crazy, but my illness is my benefactor."

The added bonus of a daily ration of whiskey prescribed by Dr. Daniel gave Jock more than a measure of pleasure. And Jock savored that whiskey from a crystal glass, a gift from Brian.

Seafaring Stories

One day Head Nurse Claire shared a pleasurable afternoon of camaraderie with Jock, the sea captain, and Brian.

Jock sat facing the captain, while Brian unfurled a map of the west coast of Scotland. Both Jock and Brian bent over the map as Jock traced the small towns and villages along the Scottish coast of Argyll.

As he moved his fingers over the map, Jock painted a scene of the majestic Firth of Clyde, a river that is more like an inland sea. And as if by magic and the creative power of their minds, the three men stepped aboard the Caledonian MacBrayne Ferry on sail through the Kyles of Bute for the port at Tighnabruaich. There, Nell, the fisherwoman, waited with her oak-smoked kippers for sale. After the ferry eased its way into port, Nell, tall and strong, helped lift the gangway into place. And as the ferry passengers dismounted she sold them her oak-smoked kippers.

Jock savored the memory of those kippers as he told Brian

and the captain, "Those kippers were the finest in the entire world." He remembered how the kippers were so popular that within ten minutes of the ferry docking, Nell sold out. And she was full of apologies that her husband had not smoked enough for all the ferry passengers to share.

Jock added, "I loved those kippers. Always ordered four pairs at a time. Aye, they were grand. Mind you, I couldnae stomach them now."

"Well," said Brian, "at least you've got some wonderful memories of them."

The captain sunk back on his pillow and with the hint of a smile said, "Memories are precious. That's what keeps us going." And with those words he fell into a deep and peaceful sleep.

Brian turned to Jock. "My gramps served in the Merchant Navy during the last World War. He probably knows the west coast of Scotland, the river Clyde. Countless ships were built on the Clyde."

"Aye," Jock agreed, "he might well know the Lady Rose. Built in Glasgow in 1937. She still sails up the Alberni Inlet with freight for small villages along the coast of British Columbia. She's a lifesaver for those people, she is, she links them tae the mainland."

Brian told Jock how his gramps got him interested in charts and maps, how Gramps had taught him as a little boy to read charts. How when his gramps traced the course of the sea-faring ships, for the young Brian it was just like embarking on some wonderful adventure.

Claire listened as Brian asked Jock about his work on the Bowen Queen, a ferry that carries cars and passengers to and from Bowen Island every day.

Jock joked lightly, "My work on the Bowen Queen was mainly to pack in as many cars and trucks as possible. So if you'd looked doon from the passenger deck onto the car deck, you might think you'd opened up a can of sardines. Mind you, naebody waits on Bowen wae prize kippers for sale."

When the head nurse left their room to complete her patient visits, the pleasant voices of both men followed her down the hallway until fading away. And she mused over the power and healing balm of camaraderie and stories shared.

"Pain as big as the universe"

Palliative care is not and never can be an individual pursuit. Palliative care is about community.

A Vietnamese Family at Dunira

The emergency light above Mr. Tee's bed signaled his distress. In trembling, broken English, the newly admitted Mr. Tee tried to tell the nurse of his pain. Marty, the night nurse, listened but could not understand his words. Clearly he was wracked with agony, but Marty could not reach him. She knew nothing of his language, his customs, and his worldview. Marty struggled to make sense of his words, but lost in another culture, another land, she could not decipher them. All she knew was that he was Vietnamese and in pain. His grievous lamentations were clearly recognizable. But the full anguish of this small, frail man would only come to light through the help and understanding of a very special sage.

The sage of understanding appeared in the form of a multicultural social worker. Summoned to his beside, she worked with the small, frail man, despite the early-morning hour. She translated his alarming words, and this is what Mr. Tee said: "My pain is as big as the universe. It's a big finger boring into my soul. Soon I will die. Please help me!"

Marty gave him morphine and waited at his side until the morphine reached his pain. Mr. Tee closed his eyes. His breathing relaxed and Marty tiptoed back to her desk to write notes on the magnitude of Mr. Tee's pain.

But where does one begin to ease the suffering of another?

Nurse Marty could not comprehend "pain as big as the universe" and suffering that "bore into the soul." No matter how compassionate, there is not a single person who can experience the suffering of another. But Marty acknowledged the essence and the integrity of this critically ill man and indicated her willingness to embrace his suffering.

Mr. Tee's problems were of such magnitude that he required the services and resources of those who understood his language and his culture. Marty called for ongoing consultation with the multicultural social worker. Her skills as a mediator, translator, and advocate included support for Mr. Tee's wife and two schoolboy sons. Like others in the community whose native tongue was not English, the services of a multicultural social worker provided a lifeline of advocacy and friendship in times of need. And Mr. Tee and his family were in desperate need.

Minh, a Boy Made Old Before His Time

Mr. Tee's fourteen-year-old son, Minh, had taken on the enormous responsibility of caring for both his parents and his ten-year-old brother. At the onset of his father's illness, Minh left his innocence behind. He was weighed down with problems far beyond his age. For one so young to be plagued with worries, to face the ultimate crisis in life, to conceal his own suffering, and to conduct himself in the manner of a grown man, was the measure of Minh's courage and selfless integrity.

Yet despite these sacrifices Minh would ultimately be labeled an angry dropout because of truancy from school.

By assuming the role of his father's protector, Minh had convinced himself that he was the one person who understood the nature and degree of his father's suffering. This belief led Minh to insist that he attend each and every hospice meeting that discussed his father's care. Dr. Daniel welcomed Minh's insight and participation, for the wisdom that Minh shared eased his father's heavy burden. Without a doubt Minh had become his father's second skin.

Mr. Tee's life resembled the broken pieces of a puzzle—a puzzle that lay strewn and scattered in many directions. Emigration to Canada severed the ties that bound him to his homeland. Uprooted from the land of his birth and not yet assimilated into the culture of Canada, Mr. Tee and his family were overwhelmed by the trauma of illness. Illness changed the shape of life and living for Mr. Tee and his dependents. The future was bleak, full of broken dreams, worries, and unmet expectations.

Mr. Tee knew that he would not live to see his two sons grow into manhood. And death would reveal a guilty secret. Mr. Tee had remortgaged the family home to pay off debts from gambling. His death would leave the family homeless, because there was no insurance to cover mortgage costs and no money to provide an income for his family. There was not even enough money to cover his burial.

In the early days of her husband's admission to Dunira, Mrs. Tee knew nothing of these facts that "bore into her husband's soul." She was not aware of the source of his torment. Mr. Tee had not shared this private hell with his wife.

Mrs. Tee worked in a laundromat. Her hours were long, her wages low. Long hours of labor left her little time to care for her two schoolboy sons. Once again, Minh jumped into the breach to nurture and set the rules of conduct for his younger brother.

With no knowledge of Minh's grim reality, the staff at Minh's school hung a label round his neck that marked him as an undesirable, angry dropout. The label was unwarranted. Indeed it was intolerant and cruel. To understand the nature of Minh's truancy from school and grasp the meaning of his anger required looking beyond the obvious to uncover deeper truths. School staff was unaware that Minh's parenting of his parents, and his time spent at Dunira Hospice, left him no time to attend school or take care of his own needs.

A Committed Hospice Team

The problems confronting this Vietnamese family were like shifting sands that required continuous adjustment in the provision of patient and family care. Countless hours were spent in the coordination and provision of services for the Tees. The daunting task of eliminating problems and providing support for the entire family required the combined forces of two social workers. The multicultural social worker and Dunira's social worker worked together to set in motion a network of essential social services for the well-being of the Tee family.

Nonetheless, Mrs. Tee bore the appearance of a woman on the verge of collapse as worry, anger, and grief bore down on her. She was overwhelmed by her husband's illness and unable to care for her two young sons.

They were a family in terrible crisis, a family in pain. And they required organized consultation and collaboration with a full network of medical and social services, including:

- Office of the Public Trustee

- Public Health Services

- Social Welfare

- Indigent Burials

- Low-Income Housing

- Grief Counseling

- Parenting Skills

- Money Management

- Nutritional Services

- School Staff

- Uncles and Aunts at Large (a mentoring service for children)

Faced with the complexities of Mr. Tee's troubled life, could anyone dispute the need for a collaborative network of medical and social services? No single individual could possibly undertake and manage the enormous problems that caused the suffering experienced by Mr. Tee and his family. No single person or service could possibly assume that they knew what was best for this patient.

It must be acknowledged that palliative care is not and never can be an individual pursuit. The impact and complex nature of catastrophic illness requires a multidisciplinary team approach. And in palliative care, a team of professional caregivers utilizes community resources in the provision of patient and family care.

Mr. Tee's pain was "as big as the universe." His psychosocial problems were overwhelming and caused him unbridled suffering. At the conclusion of Mr. Tee's life, the enormity of problems had crushed his person, leaving his family bereft, grieving, and dependent on social assistance and support.

The palliative team had reached out to the community to find the help that Mr. Tee's family so desperately needed. And the community had reached back. No doubt challenges lay ahead for Mrs. Tee and her sons, but community resources were there to help them. Just as one offers a hand to another in need, palliation lies at the heart of community.

Wayne's Fears: "Are you the worker that deals with death?"

No one ever outgrows the need
for love and understanding.

What a spectacle they made on their path of near collision. The unexpected incident occurred in Dunira's hallway. He was dressed in a back-to-front hospital gown. She was Jean, Dunira's social worker. His free arm guided the pole that supported his intravenous drip. Her free arm encircled a notepad and a human-sized teddy bear. His intravenous pole seemed to extend like some frail limb from his own wasted body. Their near collision had almost sent them both flying. From the young man's frantic expression and sunken eyes, he peered at Jean as she struggled to hold on to the plush, over-sized teddy bear. The sheer girth and height of the stuffed toy was almost larger than the young man who stood before her.

In a rushed, desperate voice, the young man blurted out, "I'm Wayne. I'm an outpatient. And I'm in for treatment. Down in Outpatients they told me to come here for grief counseling. They said you guys had some sort of group you run. This is Wednesday, isn't it? Wednesday. They said that's when the group meets."

Not stopping to catch his breath, his words ran on, almost tripping themselves with distress. "You see, uh, I'm HIV positive. And, uh, and likely I'm going to get full-blown AIDS. And downstairs they told me that up here I'd get some help. And I really need to see the 'Worker That Deals with Death.'"

A wave of shock and disbelief hit Jean. What on earth? This young man was searching the hospice for a "Worker That Deals with Death"? For one long moment she was utterly dumbstruck. How could she possibly answer such a preposterous, nonsensical question?

But he insisted, his voice turning loud and urgent. "Tell me. Are you the Worker That Deals with Death?"

For a blinding instant Jean wondered if the young man imagined her as the Fourth Horseman of the Apocalypse from the biblical prophecy in the book of Revelation.

The Fourth Horseman, or Grim Reaper, represents the scourge of death from disease, famine, wars, and violent disasters. The prophecy of the Fourth Horseman epitomizes the universal fear of death, as well as the fear that nothing in the world is permanent.

As author and journalist Andrew Nikiforuk wrote about the impact of the AIDS epidemic:

"The Fourth Horseman still rides into our lives at his convenience. AIDS offers more proof that Pestilence never rests."[10]

Illness, Isolation, and Fear

Could it be that the Grim Reaper was embedded in the minds of the staff in the Outpatients Department? Or why else had they sent a young man with death-related questions to Palliative Care in search of the "Worker That Deals with Death"? The young man had no knowledge of palliation and was almost paralyzed with fear when he walked through the door of Dunira Hospice. Yet despite his fear he had come because the isolation of his solitude was unbearable. And he was in desperate need of understanding and support.

The young man's primary objective was to locate the "Worker That Deals with Death." What an impossible idea! Just thinking about it left Jean stunned speechless, unable to think logically, unable to move. Frozen to the spot, her imagination took over. And in her mind a scene of black humor unfolded.

A caricature of the Grim Reaper—a grotesque figure riding a sleek black horse—seized Jean's imagination. Dressed in flowing black robes, the Reaper rode his powerful steed. But there was no scythe in sight. Where was his terrible scythe? It was nowhere to be found. Instead, the figure in black clasped something by its ear. What a scene! The Reaper rode past with a teddy bear in tow. The image in Jean's mind was so diabolical, so absurd, and comical, it dissolved her stress in one sudden burst.

At the image of the Grim Reaper and his teddy bear, Jean started to laugh. The laughter started low in her gut where it tumbled and gurgled, until like a cyclone it forced its way out in a delicious explosion. And Wayne was caught by its force. Jean wanted to hug this frightened young man, but as laughter seized control, she lost all physical coordination. The infectious mirth seized the two of them in its grip. And neither could stop

laughing. But it was like balm for their souls, a soothing, healing balm, and a precious moment shared.

When finally they were able to breathe again, Wayne said,
"I couldn't live without laughter. I'd go crazy without it."

Before she could speak, Jean wiped the tears of humor from
her eyes. "Sometimes," she said, "laughter is like crying inside.
But nobody knows because it comes in a different shape."

Wayne looked at Jean with glowing eyes and nodded. "Yeah.
Sometimes being an alright silly kid is the only thing to do."

Theirs had been an unusual and very close encounter in
Dunira's corridor, but at least it had put the young man at ease.

Still clutching the over-sized teddy, Jean introduced herself.
"I'm the social worker. We don't have anyone here "That Deals
with Death" because we're too busy taking care of life. And we're
certainly not in cahoots with that awful Grim Reaper. There's
just the three of us here, you, me, and Cliff, our teddy bear. He's
our group's mascot. So, welcome, Wayne. Welcome to our hospice. I'm glad you're here. Now come and join our group."

In Need of Humanitarian Care

Wayne had learned of the hospice support group from the Outpatients Department. For Dunira Hospice to receive a referral
from the Outpatients Department requesting support for a
patient was both unusual and quite amazing. Jean wondered if
the referral was finally an acknowledgment of Dunira's many
positive contributions to the community. And she wondered if
it was a sign that the hospice was finally being fully accepted
and embraced for its unique role. But what on earth had they

told Wayne? The poor young man had plucked up his courage and arrived expecting to meet with the "Worker That Deals with Death"!

Instead, what Wayne needed was to be connected with others who would share his pain because they understood. The Outpatients Department had sent to our hospice a young man, HIV positive, and in urgent need of emotional support.

Dunira's reputation was intact.[6] No longer the "new kid on the block," Dunira Hospice had become a fully integrated and specialized unit within the acute care hospital. This was progress indeed.

Wayne had come to the unit in a state of heightened anxiety. Yet he came in search of hope. To acknowledge Wayne's fear in anticipation of pain and death is to understand the meaning of suffering.

Our human condition is such that we never outgrow our need for love, security, and understanding. These needs are heightened by illness and fear. In good health or in poor health, we come together in groups and in families. We come together to be valued for who we are. By virtue of illness there is a compelling need to be connected with others. This human need does not diminish with time.

Wayne faced a bleak future. He had lost contact with his family and had endured isolation because of unreasonable fears and negative attitudes towards the presence of AIDS. Wayne's partner had died of an AIDS-related illness. Because of Wayne's knowledge of his former partner's suffering, he willingly submitted himself to the hospice in search of a support group. The palliative care group welcomed him and fostered his sense of independence and self-worth.

---

6. See the chapter, *Dunira Hospice: Rite of Passage.*

Wayne found that the support group provided him membership in a community of care. The group fully accepted him as the unique person he was, and he acknowledged this trust bestowed. Dunira's support group was not intended to provide in-depth counseling for grief, nevertheless on a few occasions counseling was arranged. The themes developed by the participants in the support group included discussions on the following subjects: role conflict, helplessness, guilt, love, giving and receiving, relationships, sharing a hospice room, letting go, healing, and hope. The camaraderie that existed within the hospice support group was invaluable. In caring for one another, members of the group fostered direction, purpose, and individual self-worth.

There are many young people like Wayne, dying from illnesses like AIDS. For these young people robbed of their future, the AIDS tragedy is a living hell. A death sentence under protest. Some AIDS patients are admitted to acute care hospitals for treatment of severe symptoms, including pneumocystis pneumonia. Young and vulnerable, many AIDS patients face a barren reality without benefit of family support. Often they are unnecessarily and unjustly isolated because of phobic fears and negative attitudes about AIDS.

At its heart, palliation is the humanistic act of caring. And through the practice of palliation we affirm, with compassion, the basic human need for love and understanding.

Wayne, who had come looking for the "Worker That Deals with Death," found instead a life-affirming community in the bosom of Dunira Hospice.

When Good Intentions Fail

"Survey the whole, nor seek slight faults to find.
Whoever thinks a faultless piece to see,
Thinks what ne'er was, nor is, nor e'er shall be."[11]
—Alexander Pope (1688–1744)

This chapter brings to light the incidences of failed intentions that caused a group of patients and their families unnecessary suffering. "Let no harm be done" was the sincere intent of their doctors. Yet three seriously ill patients were harmed and left without hope. Each patient, in turn, endured the indignity of unattended psychosocial pain. The patients' voices were unheard, their needs unmet. Those who suffered knew the system was flawed, not by intent, but by the fact that we are human and therefore imperfect.

Medical ethics, medical myths, and acute care services introduced realities that neglected the need for compassion in patient care. Our patients, Seumas O'Brian, Alfredo Valeri, and John Steele, might have said, "Yes, you named my illness and confirmed my poor prognosis. And yes, you analyzed my symptoms. But your findings did nothing to ease my suffering."

The stories of Seumas, Alfredo, and John Steele reveal that they chose to remain at home during the length of their illness. The freedom to make personal choices concerning their illness sustained them. Yet, when faced with the traumatic news of terminal illness, are vulnerable patients and their families in a position to make logical decisions that are in their own best interest? It is important to note that there was no hospice in the community where the three men resided. Nevertheless, the cottage hospital reserved three beds for palliative care patients. This fact, known to the oncologists who attended those patients, was unknown to Seumas, Alfredo, and John Steele. In hindsight, an admission to the cottage hospital would have served Alfredo well, but not the other two men.

In the community where the three men lived, there were two family doctors who were committed to palliative care. Those doctors made home visits and, in collaboration with the community palliative care team, provided patient and family care to their patients.

Medical specialists at the hospital served two masters: 1) their treatment goals of cure, and 2) the eradication of malignant tumors. When treatment failed to produce a cure, they offered palliative care.

But palliative care should not be provided on a whim or as an afterthought.

Palliative care is a serious medical commitment to relieve the pain and suffering of the terminally ill. And therefore a referral for this service requires active follow-up. But, taxed by the limitations of their resources, the oncologists did not prevail upon the health care system to establish ongoing palliative care for patients staying at home.

Dr. Bigman, senior member of the hospital staff, was an unofficial supporter of the community palliative care nurses. Notwithstanding his endorsement of palliative care, some of his patients missed the opportunity for this specialized home care service. Perhaps this oversight was related to the fact that the hospital was in a state of transition. Patients and staff were subjected to overcrowded conditions while waiting for the completion of a new facility. The community nurses had no office space within the hospital, yet they were expected to conduct sensitive patient and family interviews for newly referred palliative patients. Late patient referrals delayed the process and increased the distress of the seriously ill.

Seumas, Alfredo, and John Steele were all dependent on their families for ongoing support, acceptance, and care. Perhaps with the benefit of hindsight and the support of those whom they trusted, those patients and their families would have altered the course of events and circumstances that changed their lives. Within their stories lies a wisdom that illuminates the meaning of illness and points to possible solutions for the alleviation of patient suffering.

John Steele's Story

Nurse Beth received John Steele's referral for palliative care during the late afternoon. Dr. Bigman gave Beth a summary report of Mr. Steele's medical status in preparation for the meeting. From Dr. Bigman, Beth learned of the stature of the fifty-two-year-old cattle rancher. But strangely, the summary report made no mention of the patient's wife, Lorna.

Lorna Steele's absence during this first palliative care home assessment concerned Nurse Beth because it emphasized John Steele's solitary status and isolation.

Beth met with John Steele in Dr. Bigman's office. She found him blunt and to the point. And in spite of the serious nature of his illness, he retained his dignity and composure.

Preoccupied with a new reality that no longer resembled his past, John Steele told Beth, "My life has no meaning. Illness has stolen my way of life. It's as if some dry prairie wind stormed in and blew away all the soil that once nurtured my land. Nothing's left. It's just a strange, barren place where broken, upturned roots have displaced the foundation of my life. Not so long ago I dreamed of sons to invest in my ranch and daughters to bring me joy. But I have neither sons, nor daughters. All my dreams for tomorrow are gone."

And right there in Dr. Bigman's small, tight office, Nurse Beth learned of the depth of John Steele's suffering.

Beth listened to the flat, hollow voice of this once able rancher. His voice filled the room with the enormity of his suffering. Thoughts and feelings hung in the air like dark uncertain clouds.

She heard John Steele say, "I come to the hospital every other week and that big man gives me a going over. But I can't bear the sight of his grim face. He's always at a loss for what to say. And now that big doctor has sent you. Why did he ask you into his office? Why does he want me to speak to you? You're a nurse and a social worker. And I don't need welfare. I can pay for what I need."

Beth leaned forward and replied, "Mr. Steele, the welfare that I offer has nothing to do with social assistance. But it has everything to do with your welfare and your well-being."

She paused a moment, then continued. "When you asked Dr. Bigman for the truth about your illness, he listened and he heard your pain."

John Steele was silent now and then he heard Beth say, "Illness is a family affair. Just as palliative care is a team affair. And when we work together as a team, we share the management of your illness. And as well as that, it's your guiding hand that tells us of your needs."

It was with dismay that Beth heard John Steele's reply.

He said, "What you offer will never work for me. And I'll tell you why."

John Steele's life review revealed a reality hitherto unseen.

Lifting his gaze to Beth, he continued, "Like the proverb says: 'The road to Hell is paved with good intentions.' Without a doubt that saying applies to me. Dr. Bigman doesn't understand what it's like for me. So all those good intentions of his are just misplaced."

In the provision of compassionate care a full understanding of how the patient views their world is crucial, because a hopeless outlook impedes the alleviation of suffering and fosters the emergence of helpless despair.

Throughout his waking and his sleeping hours, John Steele was preoccupied with the symptoms of his illness and the weakness in his legs.

He told Beth, "I can't walk the length of myself without this mechanical aide."

No longer able to fulfill his former role of husband and manager of his ranch, John Steele's world lay crumbled at his feet. He saw himself a broken, crippled man who stood alone and defeated, observing life as it passed him by.

BLOCKED COMMUNICATION

Nurse Beth listened to John Steele's story and heard him say, "Before I lost my health, my wife showed not one bit of interest in the ranch. It's only now I realize that we've gone our separate ways. But if I'm truthful, I know it's always been like that. Why didn't I see it earlier? Lorna and me have been marching to different drums for years. Could it be that now she wants revenge? She looks at me with pity. She doesn't look at me like I'm a man. She excludes me from all the discussions about the ranch. She's running everything with my assistant manager. It's like I don't even exist. It's such cruel irony. Cruel, cruel irony. My wife is killing me with kindness. Her mothering is smothering me! God knows she has emasculated me. She treats me like some pathetic child."

He paused a moment, then turned with pleading eyes to Beth. "Will you talk to Lorna? Will you tell her that a man can't live like this?"

Illness is an indignity that is shared by family members and significant others. Prolonged illness places a heavy burden of responsibility on families. At times, family relations are strained to their limit of endurance. Illness may also strengthen the bond of care between patient and family. Without a doubt, illness measures and tests the strength of human relationships. In caring for a person who is ill, communication is of utmost importance. Open communication between patient and caregiver is a liberating comfort.

A FAMILY IN PAIN

Illness had eroded the relationship between John and Lorna Steele. Theirs was a household divided in conflict, misunderstanding, and pain. In their large, imposing house, John and Lorna Steele occupied separate apartments. And from their private quarters, they led separate lives. Their friends mistakenly believed that John and Lorna had it all, for they had wealth beyond their needs. Their friends were unaware that John was seriously ill and no longer able to find meaning in his life. The suffering this caused consumed him.

Lorna Steele told Nurse Beth, "You can see the plight John's in. He keeps falling down. And when I try to help him, he explodes. But nobody seems to care. I can't keep John safe. He needs someone with him all the time. John's black moods and impatience are more than I can bear. At times he looks as if he hates me and that's really scary. Managing the ranch is not my thing. But John ignores my efforts. Why can't he understand that I'm not one of his ranch hands? I do the best I can. But no matter what I do, it's never good enough. I can't go on like this. I have no peace of mind. Do you hear what I'm saying? Can you imagine how awful this whole thing is?"

LOSS OF INDEPENDENCE AND CHOICES REMOVED

Lorna Steele did not understand the nature of palliative care. She condemned it out of hand and refused palliative home care for her husband. She was preoccupied only with preventing John's frequent falls, and was unaware of his shame and loss of independence. Acting as both guardian and custodian, Lorna hired round-the-clock private care for her husband.

In medical emergencies when life hangs in the balance, round-the-clock care is appropriate. But John did not require acute intensive care. John sought compassionate understanding and autonomy in decisions that affected his life. For John, palliation would have offered the hope that his participation in the management of his illness would restore his dignity as an independent, thinking person.

Instead, John was subjected to personal private care that was custodial and enforced his dependency. Such autocratic control smacks of paternalism, which is contrary to the principles of palliative care because it exacerbates suffering. As an expression of his helpless resignation, John neither responded to, nor rejected, the round-the-clock care.

What responsibility do caregivers bear for the suffering of John and Lorna Steele? Why did they not intervene and inform Lorna of the erosion of her husband's self-esteem? A neurological explanation from Dr. Bigman about the cause and loss of her husband's mobility would have offered Lorna a more expansive view of her husband's illness. But no such explanation was given. Nor was it sought.

Lorna Steele had no understanding that the greater problem facing her husband was his loss of hope and the devastation of his noninvolvement in decisions that affected his life.

Yet awareness and understanding of another's suffering is a forward step in eradicating painful problems.

Sadly, the personal affairs of this husband and wife obscured Dr. Bigman's medical view. Perhaps Dr. Bigman was simply overwhelmed with a problem not of his making. Still, the doctor tried to bridge the gap that divided this husband and wife, but his attempts failed because it was beyond his scope to heal the hurts and wounds of a fractured marriage.

RESIGNATION AND CAPITULATION

Regarding the provision of palliative home care, John Steele had previously told Nurse Beth, "What you offer will never work for me. And I'll tell you why."

John then proceeded to share selected passages from his *Book of Life*. His story revealed his loss of selfhood and the solitude of his isolation. Nurse Beth learned about the struggles of this dignified man and yearned to help him. But Lorna's rejection of palliative services for John at home was intractable. Just as intractable was John's resignation and capitulation to Lorna's round-the-clock private care. Nurse Beth was left with a deep sense of failure at her inability to help this man in desperate need.

John Steele's private caregivers kept him from falling down. But in protecting him, they robbed him of his manhood and his freedom—a precious gift denied.

Round-the-clock hired help is obtained at considerable cost. Yet wealth does not alleviate suffering, nor does it restore dignity to the person who is seriously ill. To deny a person's choice in decisions related to the management of his or her care is to remove any vestige of hope.

The relationship between John and Lorna had long festered into a deep, irreparable wound. John, once a strong, capable rancher who ran his beloved ranch with ease, had lost control of everything that gave meaning to his life. Lorna, once a dependent wife who had busied herself with hobbies outside of the ranch, suddenly found herself thrust into the management of a ranch for which she held no interest. John and Lorna's roles had reversed, and not by choice. This reversal of roles was capped by a working relationship between Lorna and the assistant manager to run the ranch, a working relationship that excluded John.

Lorna's rejection of palliation for her husband, and John's acquiescence, was due to a lack of understanding of the benefits of such care. Instead, Lorna believed she simply needed to protect her husband from his falls. But her attempts to rescue John reduced him to the status of a crippled child, which only fueled his rage. And Lorna could make no sense of the rage directed at her every attempt to protect her husband and hold the ranch together.

Inevitably, the transitions fostered by serious illness upend our lives and challenge our roles within them. These upheavals are worsened by the same ingredients that sow disharmony: an unhappy marriage, a lack of understanding and communication, a loss of identity, dignity, and hope, a lack of tenderness and love.

It takes time to right the wrongs of unmet expectations in roles that are reversed, of triangulation and separation. But time is relentless as it marches on. And despondency and hopelessness can hasten death's approach.

THE EXACERBATION OF SUFFERING

In the final stages of his illness, John Steele was confined to his own private quarters. Never left alone, his protective ever-watchful caregivers became his well-meaning and kindly jailers. Resting on his leather couch, John Steele acknowledged that for him there was no moving forward. His past was gone, and he could not reclaim it. Unable to walk, John Steele had become a bedridden invalid who suffered the indignity of a drug-induced state of oblivion.

In his need to escape the boredom and burden of the sameness of every day, John Steele used the power of his creative mind and claimed his one remaining choice. His final decision gave him unending peace. There was one who would carry him away. She was steadfast and willing and would carry him on her back. Once again in the spirit of freedom he would breathe the air of the sweet green plains, relish the wide blue canopy of sky over his beloved open range. And so, in his mind, John Steele took up the reigns of his steadfast little mare and quickly rode away.

The Story of Seumas

It could be said of Seumas that he denied being ill. Visits to the hospital were an imposition he would gladly forgo. Some might consider him fearful and judge the denial of his illness as a negative force in his life. Others might ask if denial served a purpose.

Is denial a human defense against a hopeless situation? Are laughter and denial a way to cope with life's ultimate crises?

> "Most human beings have the capacity for coming to terms with their circumstances, which they retain even as death approaches, though for some it is a struggle that is deeply painful to watch. Others appear to hold quite contradictory feelings in an uneasy balance."[12]

Seumas made denial his companion. And denial was the companion that eased his fear of dying.

Supported by his loving family, Seumas found no need to go in search of medical truths from his cancer specialist, Dr. Ethic. Instead, Seumas preferred half-truths laced with humor. He saw humor in most things and with the skill of an artist he used myth and humor to erase his pain.

Kathleen said of her husband, "Seumas missed his calling, for surely he has the gift of the gab. My Seumas is full of the blarney, and wherever there is laughter, Seumas is in its midst. A beautiful man, he is my strong right arm."

Seumas loved life. At forty-two years young, he braved each day, ignoring the tumor that grew inside his head. Seumas gave no credence to the shadows that dimmed his eyes for he believed in the power of positive thinking. For Seumas, there was no room for calamity.

Kathleen, devoted wife of Seumas, when laughter has fled the scene and weeping and grieving mark the time of unwanted change, will you hold your man with your two strong arms and protect him from harm? For that day draws near, and grim it will be when denial of his illness no longer comforts Seumas.

Seumas did not wish to be told that he was seriously ill, nor that a tumor would deprive him of his life. There were times when he heard the wisdom of his mind. And it warned him, *Something's wrong.*

But Seumas denied the logic of his common sense. And with the dawn of each new day, he ignored his fatigue and the headaches that ensued.

DR. ETHIC'S HONORABLE INTENTIONS

Dr. Ethic examined the chart that lay open on his desk. The chart belonged to Seumas and it revealed a tumor that chemotherapy had failed to restrain. The doctor's findings were grim. It was the doctor's responsibility to inform the patient of his medical prognosis and the failure of the treatment. Without question, patients have the right to be informed of their medical status.

Doctors are continually faced with difficult problems affecting their patients' lives. However, regardless of ethics, moral responsibilities, and honorable intentions, medical information must always be given with cautious sensitivity.

Compassionate patient care is a partnership that invites communication and considers the patient a person of unique personality and social identity, with his or her own hopes and dreams. It is crucial to be aware of the patient's readiness and/or ability to tolerate bad news.

It is foolhardy to proceed with detailed medical information, especially when a seriously ill patient has made no such request of their doctor. For such information is likely to instill a sense of dread that erodes all hope.

When cure is no longer possible, the wise, compassionate doctor invites confirmation of their patients' needs by listening to their stories. Then without haste, the doctor answers any questions that may be asked. Through the simple, humanistic act of sharing, the doctor confirms the continuation of comfort care and support for their seriously ill patients.

Dr. Ethic considered the positive aspects of the medical information he planned to share with Seumas. He believed that given the facts of his untreatable illness, Seumas would have the opportunity to settle his personal affairs and put his house in order. And that, in and of itself, was positive.

But Seumas had never asked the oncologist about his medical progress. Seumas was in denial; he had never asked because he did *not* want to be told that he was dying. Therein lies a dilemma that becomes a source of patient harm. For some patients, the impact of such a grim prediction leads to early demise. Such was the case for Seumas.

Dr. Ethic's knowledge of Seumas was encapsulated in the microscopic view of an untamed tumor. He had no knowledge of Seumas the man, no knowledge of the humanity and passion of Seumas the person. In fact, Dr. Ethic had no knowledge of how Seumas would receive any news that concerned his illness.

Seumas was unaware that this one meeting with Dr. Ethic would mark his final visit to the hospital. Unprepared and taken by surprise at the outcome of the meeting, Seumas suffered.

As was his usual practice, Dr. Ethic sat behind his large and very imposing desk. He opened a folder and silently read its contents as Seumas and Kathleen sat respectfully, waiting quietly for the doctor's words. After a long moment, Dr. Ethic looked up, looked Seumas straight in the eye, and delivered his medical prognosis.

Seumas heard only twenty percent of what the doctor said. But that twenty percent came in the darkest possible shade of black. Seumas heard only the words, "Your cancer is on the rampage. It's out of control. I'm sorry. There's nothing more we can do."

Dr. Ethic paused before saying, "At most, I'll give you six more weeks."

How those words took hold of Seumas. They burned inside

his head, carving pictures seen only in nightmares. In shock, Seumas heard the pronouncement of his own death sentence, "*six more weeks,*" from a doctor, a specialist, who knew all the answers. Surely the doctor was right. Surely his doctor's predictions would come to pass.

Grim were Dr. Ethic's words. Grim was his prognosis. Seumas was left without hope.

Overcome with passion and with a force that surprised even himself, Seumas jumped up, grabbed the nearest chair, raised it to his chest, and holding the chair in his two strong hands, Seumas swiftly broke its back. Splinters of the broken chair flew around the room.

The force of Seumas's reaction rendered Dr. Ethic speechless. Immediately the doctor understood the consequence and impact of the "medical truth" he had just shared. In that same instant he also realized how he had failed to consider the anguish and passion of Seumas the person. And how in that failing he had only exacerbated Seumas's suffering.

Now Dr. Ethic heard Seumas yelling, "Good God, man. I asked you for nothing. I sure as Hell didnae ask you for that."

All that Seumas had heard in the doctor's "medical truth" was the clanging of a persistent bell. The clanging bell took its toll and marked the time of his death.

Oh what power language has, especially words that take no account of their impact, their crushing force. Words, like tumbling boulders, can kill all living hope.

In his haste to tell his patient that there was no cure, Dr. Ethic did not stop to listen or consider the impact of his words. Ethical concerns and honorable intentions had gotten in the doctor's way and obscured his patient's point of view.

It is *not* possible to predict time of death. Such predictions are at best an educated guess based on statistical information. Should not the mystery and time of death be left in the hands of nature?

Following the episode of the broken chair, Dr. Ethic hastened to make amends to Seumas by offering palliative care. But given the circumstances, Seumas was in no mood for further talk. Seumas was in a state of shock and could not hear the benefits of palliation.

Although Dr. Ethic proposed that Seumas and Kathleen receive continued care, this offer of palliation followed his statement that, "There's nothing more we can do."

Surely that was a contradiction. For one might ask, what does palliation offer if "There is nothing more we can do"?

It is cruel nonsense to claim that nothing can be done. There is *always* something that can be done to support, comfort, and improve the quality of care for a patient who is terminally ill.

Summoned by Dr. Ethic's referral for palliative care, Beth, the palliative nurse, witnessed the pale, quivering shock of both Seumas and Kathleen. The couple sat huddled together in the clinic lounge overwhelmed by an immense and private world of grief. And in that ragged state of sorrow and trauma, all Nurse Beth could do was to offer them her outstretched hand, then quietly drive them home. At times, the kindest, most compassionate thing to do is to acknowledge the suffering of others by being fully present and respectfully silent.

Kathleen and Seumas left that fearful place consumed by troubled thoughts. Let no one intrude, for their grief was raw, unspeakable, and beyond the comprehension of others.

A FAMILY AFFAIR

Two weeks passed with no news of Seumas.

Nurse Beth's first visit to Seumas and Kathleen's home was an unexpected and startling experience. Kathleen opened the front door wide with the words, "Come away in, Beth. You'll be wanting a word with Seumas. He's waiting for you in the front room."

Nurse Beth entered the room at the front of the house and was taken by surprise. The room was filled with people and there in their midst stood Seumas. Was it not always so that Seumas would gather together his friends? For all of life and living was worthy of a grand celebration and nothing less would do!

Dressed in his fine dark suit, wearing a white shirt and black tie, Seumas appeared to be standing amidst the group, silent, without voice, unable to speak his welcome. It was only then that Beth saw that Seumas was dead, propped upright to attend his own untimely wake. His fire and passion had gone, but the memory and joy of Seumas remained.

This was Nurse Beth's first experience of a wake, and it taught her the value of this celebration. The wake is a memorial, an acceptance, and a preparation for change. By restoring memories of the deceased, it bestows respect and eases the pain of grief.

Music and poetry, love and laughter were the essence of Seumas. And so they came in honor of Seumas, their passionate Gael. Seumas would surely have approved of the gathering that encircled him. For the gathering was a coming together, a rallying point and social ritual for family and friends. It was a ritual of acceptance and gratitude for the joy that was Seumas's life. A ritual that enabled each and every one to frame their lives. And all who filled that room joined together to honor the memory of Seumas. Through stories, music, and verse, friends and family paid their respects.

United in a joyous celebration, Seumas was sent on his journey to the hereafter. With outstretched hands, they clasped one another in a circle and together sang a Gaelic song. The ringing sound of the song's words filled the hearts of everyone in that circle. For the words of the song were full of grace and meaning, a tribute of farewell to Seumas, a humanist and a Gael: "Goodnight and joy be with you."

Alfredo's Story

Sofia, wife of Alfredo, if along the way you met your fellow travelers, John and Lorna Steele, Seumas and Kathleen, what gift of wisdom would you have shared? Their pain was overwhelming, yet it was pain you understood. For you had suffered and endured, as you lovingly applied the salve to ease your husband's wounds. There was never any question in your mind, Sofia, that home and family filled your husband's needs, for well you knew that illness is and has always been a family affair.

At the onset of his illness at the age of fifty-two, Alfredo found comfort in the caring ministrations of his wife. She was his confidant, his shaman, and his healer all in one. And she openly shared the experience of her husband's illness.

Dr. Fred was Alfredo's palliative care physician and family doctor. His patients knew the doctor as a caring family man. Dr. Fred worked long hours, made home visits, found time for humor, and loved all things Italian. He was committed to the provision of palliative care within the patient's home. His frequent visits and the clarity of his communications lent support to Alfredo and his family. Many evenings, Dr. Fred was found in the company of Alfredo. And in listening to the conversation that passed between the two men, it was obvious that each found pleasure in happy recollections of boyhood adventures in Italy.

Alfredo's only request of Dr. Fred was to remain at home during his illness. Dr. Fred assured Alfredo of continued comfort care in his home. With palliative care firmly in place, Dr. Fred assured Alfredo that he would not suffer undue pain from illness.

Sofia, Dr. Fred, and the palliative nurses became Alfredo's able and caring team. From Nurse Beth, Sofia learned the importance of Alfredo's four-hourly pain medicine. And Alfredo always received his day and night medicine on time.

Despite having no formal training in health care, Sofia established a miniature hospice for Alfredo's continued care. Taught by Nurse Beth, Sofia learned how to observe the quality of her husband's pain. She learned to distinguish the difference between chronic and acute pain. Nurse Beth gave the example of acute pain as the kind of pain that follows surgery that is of short duration and ends when healing takes place. In contrast, chronic pain is continuous.

Advanced tumor pain is chronic and its management requires informed knowledge of pain's occurrence, what heightens the pain, and what relieves it. A restless, anxious state signals the presence of pain. The palliative management of chronic cancer pain seeks to achieve an alert, comfortable patient who is relatively pain-free.

Alfredo suffered chronic neurological pain related to a malignant brain tumor. But during the time Alfredo remained at home, he was relaxed and comfortable. His comfortable state was achieved through ongoing assessment of his pain, and recorded observations of his mood, sleep, and ability to communicate with caregivers. Thus a profile of Alfredo's state of being was established and resulted in a pain regimen of four-hourly oral morphine. At times, his pain medications required adjustment or titration, increasing or reducing, the dose of morphine in order to maintain his level of comfort.

Resting in his big reclining chair, Alfredo was included in the hub of family life. And in the security and comfort of his home he listened with joy to the classical music of the old maestros. Sofia told Nurse Beth, "Alfredo's music helped our two sons grow."

Sofia's Italian hospitality, her laughter, and delicious coffee crème lightened the workload of her husband's palliative team. There were times when the English language baffled Sofia, yet she knew the meaning and nature of compassion. She understood that hospice is a seven-letter word at the root and core of the word hospitality. And Sofia's hospitality extended a welcome to all those who entered her home.

Alfredo's choice to remain at home was honored by his wife and Dr. Fred, his trusted doctor. At home, Alfredo was in a safe and loving environment. And that was the environment where he should have remained to live each day surrounded by family and the music he loved. But a nightmare of events intruded and took their toll, shattering Alfredo's hospitable world. It started with the diabolical force of a grand-mal seizure. Then everything changed.

SOFIA'S DILEMMA

Sofia experienced Alfredo's severe epileptic seizure with terror. Never before had she seen anyone in the grip of a convulsive fit, let alone a grand-mal seizure. Alfredo was cyanosed, dark blue in color, and Sofia thought that he was dead. Alone, blinded by panic, she tried without success to reach Dr. Fred. Instead, her emergency call reached an unknown doctor whose response was immediate. Sofia was in a state of shock when the emergency doctor arrived. And in that state of shock she was unable to fully comprehend the information that he gave her.

The horror of Alfredo's near-death experience had paralyzed Sofia with fear. As if on automatic pilot, she followed the new doctor's instructions and obeyed his orders. She was told that her husband could no longer remain at home because he required hospital care, observation, and seizure-control medications. Unable to consider the implications of Alfredo's admission to an acute care hospital, Sofia agreed with the new doctor. Alfredo was immediately taken by ambulance to High Cross Hospital.

The following morning, when Nurse Beth pulled up to park her old green Land Rover outside Sofia's front door, she was struck by an eerie feeling at the strangely quiet house. Somehow the house no longer looked familiar. Once inside, she understood the reason. At the sight of Sofia, Nurse Beth was so startled her breath caught in her throat. Sofia bore all the signs of someone deeply traumatized by grief.

Sofia's voice faltered as she spoke. "I am to blame. I should never listened to emergency doctor. But I thought Alfredo dead."

Bewildered, Nurse Beth asked, "Sofia, tell me what happened. Where is Alfredo?"

"I should phoned you, Beth. You would told me what to

do. I needed Dr. Fred. But he away. I should never listened to emergency doctor. But Alfredo not breathing. He was jerking and choking and mouth full of foam. I didn't know what to do." Sofia's voice shook, then she burst into sobs. "I thought my Alfredo dead."

"Sofia, where is Alfredo now?"

"In hospital."

Nurse Beth took hold of Sofia's cold hands and warmed them in her own. Then she made a pot of tea, sweetened it with honey, and placed a slice of fresh ginger root in the teapot. As the two women sipped their tea, Nurse Beth learned of the catastrophic events that had occurred the previous evening.

"I hate what I done. I broke promise to Alfredo. Now I cause him more pain." Once again, Sofia repeated her anguish. "When Alfredo took fit, I got scared. It all up to me. I needed Dr. Fred. But he not there."

"Oh, Sofia," Nurse Beth said, "Dr. Fred had to rush to Italy. His father is very ill. I'm not sure when he'll be back again."

"I can't believe I let ambulance take my Alfredo," Sofia continued. "He only fifty when got that tumor in head. And make him so ill. But I promise Alfredo he stay home with me. And Dr. Fred say yes. But emergency doctor came, tell me Alfredo not stay here 'cause he need 'observation.' But what good about 'observation'? Now Alfredo all mixed up. He got so much pain."

Nurse Beth offered to phone the High Cross Hospital for news of Alfredo. The information she received from Alfredo's hospital nurse was guarded and not reassuring. Nurse Beth was told, "The patient is as well as can be expected." Such a familiar statement. But what did it mean?

Nurse Beth tried to console Sofia. "You are not to blame

for Alfredo's admission to the hospital. You were faced with a life-threatening crisis and you placed your trust in the doctor. Dr. Emerge took command and you followed his instructions. But you need to know that High Cross Hospital is an acute care facility. It doesn't offer palliative care. And since Dr. Emerge admitted Alfredo to the hospital, he is now in charge of Alfredo's care. Now it is Dr. Emerge who will determine the treatment and medication orders for Alfredo."

In consideration of the circumstances that led to Alfredo's hospital admission, Nurse Beth wondered how many of us would claim no regrets for decisions made in the grip of a fearful life crisis.

ACUTE PATIENT CARE IS NOT PALLIATION

Admission to High Cross Hospital deprived Alfredo both of palliative care and the peaceful comfort and security of his home. And Sofia's attempts to improve her husband's hospital care met with the disapproval of hospital staff. Tension between Sofia and hospital staff mounted. And Alfredo suffered the consequences.

Alfredo occupied a single room next to the nursing station on the Neurological Unit. On this unit his world was no longer familiar or secure. As if nameless, he was regarded by his caregivers, not as a person, but as a series of complicated, neurological symptoms. Alfredo's pain was mismanaged and out of control. And yet the nature of his pain was fully documented in his palliative care pain regimen. The palliative management of Alfredo's pain had been developed through meticulous assessment of his illness during the many months he had spent at home under the care of his wife, his doctor, and the palliative nurses.

On admission to High Cross Hospital, Dr. Emerge replaced Alfredo's pain regimen with a *pro re nata* (prn, or as-needed) prescription of hypodermic morphine to be given if necessary or as required. But a prn doctor's order for the relief of advanced tumor pain is inappropriate, vague in meaning, and invites the possibility that the medication will not be given when it is required. Furthermore, prn prescriptions for pain seldom stand alone and are usually combined with other analgesics for the relief of acute pain.

Cancellation of Alfredo's palliative care regimen indicated that Dr. Emerge lacked knowledge in the care of a fatally ill patient with unremitting pain. The doctor's prn order for Alfredo was further proof of his lack of knowledge.

Chronic pain cannot be managed by the interpretation of others, nor can it be based solely on the assumptions or value judgments of caregivers.

"PAIN IS WHAT THE PATIENT SAYS IT IS"

> *"Pain is what the patient says it is and not what the physician expects it to be or thinks it ought to be."*[13]

Alfredo was gravely ill and no longer capable of asking for pain relief. His pain was out of control. Suffering now became Alfredo's chaotic reality.

The pain monograph states that:

Never prn
Continuous pain requires continuous analgesics. The aim of therapy is to prevent the resurgence of pain rather than to repeatedly treat it. This anticipation breaks the vicious cycle of pain—despair—more pain, which causes dose escalation. Waiting for pain to reappear, as with 'as required,' 'on demand,' or 'prn' narcotic orders is illogical and cruel and perpetuates the fear and memory of pain. While 'prn' narcotic orders may be needed for 'breakthrough' pain, the basis of control must be regular scheduling."[14]

Aware of her husband's unremitting pain, Sofia's anxiety grew. She felt powerless to relieve Alfredo's suffering. Sofia knew that the nursing staff on this specialized unit misunderstood her. There was no meaningful communication or consultation between Sofia and the hospital staff. Instead, Sofia was held at arm's length by the acute care nurses, who thought she was hysterical. The silence of the hospital staff increased Sofia's guilt about Alfredo's admission to the hospital. And the dying Alfredo was denied the comfort of his family's personal care.

Driven by anger and despair, Sofia approached the nursing station to report on Alfredo's suffering. She was determined to achieve her objective when she demanded morphine for Alfredo. But her demands to relieve her husband's pain fell on deaf ears. Instead, Sofia was admonished.

As Sofia stamped her foot on the hard linoleum floor, she informed Alfredo's nurse of her husband's restless, confused state. Sofia knew that her husband's agitated state was an indication of uncontrolled pain.

The nurse responded in the dismissive tone of authority. "Mrs. Valeri, your husband's restlessness is symptomatic of a malignant brain tumor. And you are not authorized to dictate the administration of a narcotic for your husband."

"Can't you see Alfredo in agony?" Sofia cried in urgent protest. "What good all your observations? The only thing I get from you, words, words, repeat, repeat. Nothing for comfort to my poor Alfredo."

A near-hysterical Sofia continued to stamp her foot, as once again she demanded morphine for her husband. Sofia refused to leave the nursing station. Her angry outburst led the nurses to perceive her as a bossy, interfering woman. So they called security.

Sofia endured the utmost humiliation when hospital security unceremoniously escorted her to the door. For Sofia, there was no dignity, only shame and misery. But the ultimate victim in this shockingly tragic scenario was Alfredo the patient, who was rendered helpless and left in unremitting pain.

In one nightmarish sequence of events, Alfredo's grand mal seizure had resulted in the loss of his palliative home care. His life had been threatened by the occurrence of the seizure and indicated a need for seizure-control medication. But his emergency admission to the acute care hospital ended the provision of his palliative care pain regimen and rendered him helpless without dignity or hope.

Instead, an admission of Alfredo to one of the palliative care beds at the cottage hospital would have been more appropriate and should have taken place. Seizure-control medicine, including Alfredo's palliative pain regimen, would have been accepted and implemented. Although Dr. Fred was not in attendance, the doctor's medical directives and knowledge of Alfredo would have been respectfully honored. One further benefit of a palliative admission to the cottage hospital would have been to offer respite and support to Sofia.

But sadly Alfredo remained on the Neurological Unit of an acute care hospital, where he was isolated and his pain out of control.

In recounting the situation of Alfredo's hospital stay, not only is it apparent that the physicians and nurses in acute care lacked knowledge in the fundamentals of chronic tumor pain management, they also lacked knowledge and understanding of suffering families, whose indispensable role in the provision of compassion and patient comfort was ignored. After his admission to the acute care hospital, Alfredo's suffering was magnified.

Ethical and moral responsibilities embodied in the provision of health care and moral conduct imply: *let no harm befall another.*

But harm was done to Alfredo and his family. Alfredo and Sofia were stripped of hope by a system that promised care.

When seriously ill patients lose their sense of hope they may shrivel up and die. Who will claim responsibility for the lack of compassion and loss of hope for Alfredo and his family?

Many times in her mind, Sofia visited and revisited the place where Alfredo lay helpless. Hospital staff moved around in ghoulish gowns with stethoscopes dangling from their necks. And in that maze of hospital high technology, families were displaced.

Sofia did not understand the unwritten rule of hospital etiquette that reinforces professional boundaries and excludes family involvement in patient treatment and care. Sofia never understood why the hospital denied Alfredo "proper medicine and compassionate care." Yet Sofia's gentle, personal care would have reassured Alfredo and reduced his isolation and his fear.

Alfredo did not return home. Four days following his admission to the acute care hospital, he died. His family suffered inconsolable grief.

Some weeks following the death of Alfredo, Sofia received a visit from Nurse Beth. Sofia's son showed the nurse into the living room where his mother sat silently on the floor next to Alfredo's big chair. A black shawl draped around Sofia's shoulders revealed her shrunken form. She looked much older than her forty-eight years.

Nurse Beth joined Sofia on the floor where they sat cross-legged. In a peaceful silence of unconditional love, Sofia's extended family joined them. Beth marveled at the unfolding of the soundless scene. Never before had she experienced anything like it.

In a silence full of respect, Sofia's relatives filled the room. Without announcement or ceremony, they sat in a circle close to Sofia and Nurse Beth. The feeling that filled the room was one of incomparable loving peace.

Beth felt as though she had been transported to a place where the hurts of recent yesterdays were washed away. Sofia's family members were the healers. Their respectful silence created a loving space for restoration, a fellowship of care.

As they sat together, the family asked, "Could we have prevented Alfredo's suffering? Should we have mortgaged our homes and taken him to the States for treatment?"

One by one they shared their questions, their thoughts. The warmth of one another's presence and the sharing of these precious stories comforted them. They spoke of happy memories of Alfredo's membership in a small Italian jazz band. Alfredo's memory was secure. And it felt as if Alfredo's presence filled his empty chair.

Sofia was not alone. Sofia's extended family willingly walked her way because they understood the meaning of compassion.

THE NEED FOR AWARENESS AND LEARNING

In 1985, at the first Canadian Hospice Palliative Care Conference in Winnipeg, Manitoba, Dr. Doyle, of the University of Edinburgh, Scotland, addressed the conference. He said, "It is a myth that the essentials of palliative care are taught in medicine, nursing, and other paramedical disciplines." Sadly, this remains true to this day.

Professional health care personnel attending the conference were advised of the importance and indispensable role of the family in the presence of illness.

The interdependent relationship that holds families together is fostered through the act of caring and sharing. Sofia's extended family exemplified the virtue of a close-knit caring family. Dedicated family members are a tangible link with the patient's past, present, and future.

The exclusion and intolerance of family participation in patient care deprives patients of the necessary compassion, comfort, and meaning only loved ones can offer.

If Sofia had attended this palliative care conference, she would have endorsed Dr. Doyle's statement, "It is a myth that the essentials of palliative care are taught in medicine, nursing, and other paramedical disciplines."

The time is long overdue to change this.

Hide and Seek

In the story of John Steele, four people played a game that resembled hide-and-seek. Their voices, hushed in silence, never did reveal their hiding places. Silence thwarted their efforts to be found. Out of sight and in disguise, they kept their secrets safe. No one ever knew the hidden thoughts that were locked within their minds. Yet, all the while, they waited to be found. But without commitment to one another, without a willingness to share the burden of care, all they had in common were good intentions. Good intentions that failed.

John Steele saw himself a broken man, and Lorna never understood that her mothering was "smothering" her once dynamic man. Lorna never heard her husband cry aloud, "A man can't live like this." Sadly, their communication had broken down. All that Lorna Steele could see was someone who resembled John, but he kept falling down. And so she purchased round-the-clock protection.

But the worth and dignity of a sick person cannot be purchased. The dignity of the person who is ill can only be maintained within relationships of nonjudgmental care.

At the same time, Nurse Beth and Dr. Bigman waited and observed, hoping for a miracle of change. But change comes only with consultation, cooperation, and commitment. Only then is suffering shared and understood.

In his need to escape the misery of his every single day, John Steele found his own way to leave forever his place of hiding.

Medical Myths

Following the encounter with his cancer specialist, Seumas was distressed and overcome with mortal fear.

Dr. Ethic had told Seumas, "There's nothing more that we can do. . . . I'll give you six more weeks." Palliative care was then offered to Seumas, but it followed the pronouncement of his impending death.

Given this information, whose needs were met?

Did moral conduct and ethical responsibility coupled with patient rights get in the way, removing the last fragment of hope for Seumas and Kathleen?

Or was it Dr. Ethic's myth-making prophecy that robbed Seumas of his precious hope, forcing him to face a grim reality?

No longer able to deny that he was ill, Seumas succumbed to helpless resignation.

Why do we impose our beliefs and opinions on others? After all, an opinion is not a statement of fact. An opinion is merely a conjecture of the mind, often erroneous, sometimes mere guesswork. It is a known fact that attitudes and beliefs shape our relations with others and with ourselves, as shown by the many studies on mind-body connection and the growing importance of the medical field of psychoneuroimmunology.

In addition to physical pain, many terminally ill patients suffer the anguish of fear, anger, and despair. The suffering of these patients is intensified by the attitudes of those who lack understanding of the meaning of suffering, those who manufacture myths and present them as truths.

Dr. Ethic's grim prediction deprived Seumas of all hope.

Predicting a patient's time of death can become a self-fulfilling prophecy. Seumas had the word of a specialist. And the doctor knew best. Two weeks after receiving Dr. Ethic's prediction of death, Seumas died.

Symptom Control

Alfredo was admitted to an acute care hospital as a brain-injured patient. His neurological symptoms required seizure-control medications and ongoing observation. An unfamiliar emergency doctor, who did not practice palliative care, took over Alfredo's care. As a result, Alfredo's suffering was intensified and manifestly cruel. Alfredo's pain was not managed, resulting in the chaos of ungoverned suffering, restlessness, and disorientation.

Alfredo's admission to High Cross Hospital left his wife, Sofia, isolated and disconnected. Hospital staff closed ranks against Sofia, considering Alfredo their exclusive responsibility. The staff of the Neurological Unit did not seek Sofia's wisdom regarding her husband's restless anguish. Alfredo might have been a nonentity, a mere collection of neurological symptoms that resembled a human form. Alfredo the person was no longer recognized.

Sofia was Alfredo's tangible link with his past, present, and future. She was his doctor within. Her very presence eased her husband's pain. But at High Cross Hospital, staff did not honor Sofia's ministrations to her husband. Caregivers pursued an individual approach to the habitual routine of patient care. There was no evidence of sharing, no invitation to family members to participate in the process of care. Instead, on the Neurological Unit, care consisted of doing *for* the sick and dependent.

Yet to consider doing *for* the sick and dependent *without* their participation is to negate the meaning of altruistic, interpersonal care and to forgo the art of medicine.

Hospital staff prevented Sofia from contributing to her husband's care. Yet in the world of everyday living, each of us survives in an interdependent relationship with others. It is therefore unacceptable to ignore the mutually dependent relationships that exist between people, whether they are patients, family, or caregivers. To discount the input of family in the provision of patient care is a contradiction in thinking.

Palliative care advocates for the participation of family within the hospice team. Cooperation between family, staff, and patient serves to enhance the quality of care for the seriously ill.

Many are the questions that must be asked of the staff at High Cross Hospital. It is unusual for a patient and family to receive palliative care services only to be deprived of those services at the onset of a grand mal seizure resulting in an emergency hospital admission.

Failure to provide the continuation of palliative care for Alfredo revealed errors of judgment and imperfections within the health care system. In the tragic scenario of a family in crisis and a patient in unremitting pain, who bears the responsibility for the harm that was done? Most importantly, how can we ensure that this tragic situation never happens again?

One lone voice still cries in protest, the voice of Sofia. And she asks, "Why?"

Whose Needs Are Met?

O nce I was asked if terminally ill patients and families
were better served within a hospice, such as Dunira, or if
patients and families were better served staying at home with
support from the visiting hospice team.

Palliative care services within the hospice and within the
community are the same. Palliative care is not an either-or situation; palliative services can be provided at home or in a hospice, depending on what serves the patient and family best. The
philosophy of palliative care is universal in nature and the specified goal of palliation is the alleviation of pain and suffering.

The advantages of palliative care services are well documented. In most instances, seriously ill patients and their families are given a choice of receiving home, or hospice care, and/
or some combination of both. Thus, depending on the patient
and family circumstances, and the availability of resources, the
patient's choice is honored. Family participation is a necessary
component of palliative care services.

But circumstances were clearly beyond the control of
Alfredo, Seumas, John Steele, and their families. Each of them
sought hope in the provision of compassionate patient care and
relief from "existential pain."[15] Yet hope and the alleviation of
their suffering were mismanaged and unmet.[7]

---

7. See the chapter, *When Good Intentions Fail.*

Palliative Home Care

Caring for a seriously ill person at home is demanding. And there are times when the coping capacity of families is strained to the limit of endurance. The caring presence of family and friends secures the patient's membership within their community. Family and friends link the patient with the past and the present, thus providing continuity of life.

The give-and-take of unconditional sharing and caring between family members is the glue that holds families together. In the crisis of illness, the family's cohesive strength is revealed. Caring for a seriously ill person at home can be a selfless act, requiring fortitude and, at times, respite for the families.

Palliative care is commonly provided at home, because often that is where the patient wants to be. Where possible, terminally ill patients and families are given the choice of home or hospice care and/or some combination of both, including respite hospice care.

Respite Hospice Care

Respite hospice care offers families a brief period of rest, a break from the onerous burden of continuous patient care at home. Respite care constitutes a short palliative care admission.

At Dunira, short-term patient admission resembled a short stay at a specialized health care center. Dunira's respite care was straightforward. Since all arrangements for respite were made in advance, no form-filling procedures were required at the time of admission to Dunira. During the period of respite care, the patient's needs were reassessed and, where necessary, adjustments made to pain medications. Respite care provided support and a period of rest for caring family members.

Altruism at Dunira

D unira's night nurses were weary with exhaustion. Three deaths during the night had depleted them. Sister Beatrice's early arrival on the unit brought the nurses some measure of relief from their long night and they greeted her with a smile.

Sister Beatrice sought out the senior nurse for information about Brian and Jock. Nurse Marty told Beatrice that both men had spent a sleepless night as they kept vigil at the side of the sea captain's bed. At the first light of dawn, the old captain had died.

Patient Vigils

Sister Beatrice joined Jock and Brian as they sat together in the family room.

Jock was the first to speak. "Things won't be the same now the captain's gone. Aye, we had some grand times together, we did. And I'm the richer man for knowing him."

Brian's reddened eyes told of his grief.

Sister Beatrice turned to Brian and said, "Your grandpa would tell you that it's okay to be sad. And he'd want you to finish your studies. He often told me how proud you made him feel."

By sharing her thoughts, Sister Beatrice reached out to

both of the men. "The captain sailed away this morning to meet his maker. But before leaving he shared your journey, which was more like an adventure at sea. And now you're both feeling sad because he's left you waiting on the shore—"

Before she could finish, Jock interrupted. "Aye, you're right in what you say. But it'll no be long before I join that great old man."

Altruism prevails when hospice patients refuse to change rooms because their roommate is dying. This sentiment is common. Jock shared that view and willingly remained vigilant to the end. Jock believed that to stay and care, and be present to say good-bye to his old friend, the sea captain, was the most natural thing to do.

Olga's Appeal for Help

Midmorning brought a distraught and newly widowed Olga back to Dunira Hospice. She came in search of Jean, the social worker.

Olga sat with Maria in the family room and awaited Jean's arrival. As soon as Jean rounded the corner and spotted Olga's appearance, she felt a stab of concern. Olga was shivering. Her whole body shook as if with convulsions. Jean embraced Olga, then took both of the women to her office and quietly closed the door.

Two weeks had passed since the start of Olga's bereavement. And in less than a week Olga planned to return home to the Ukraine to bury her husband.

Olga's anxious voice trembled as she told Jean, "They've lost Nick's ashes."

In disbelief, Jean asked Olga to repeat what she had said. "Stan Memorial has lost Nick's ashes. Nick was cremated. But now they've lost his remains. The director told me he would put Nick's urn in a wall niche until I was ready to take him home. How can this be? I trusted that director and look what he's done. But that fellow who answered the phone said he couldn't find Nick's ashes. What am I going to do? I'm supposed to take Nick home in four days' time. Home to the Ukraine. But now Nick's vanished. He's lost! What will his family say?"

Olga's words took Jean by surprise. A moment passed before she heard herself say, "Olga, funeral directors do not dare lose bodies. Or urns containing body remains. Such malpractice would deny them the right to serve society."

A student nurse knocked on Jean's door and asked, "Should I bring you some tea?"

Jean thanked the student, then leaned towards Olga and said, "You've had a horrible shock, Olga. A terrible mistake has been made. But rest assured, before this day is over Stan Memorial will have recovered Nick's urn and placed it safely in the wall niche. I'll arrange a time for you and me to go to Stan Memorial and we'll bring Nick home. I give you my word, Olga. And I won't let you down."

The two women left the social worker to sort out the problem with Stan Memorial. The women retreated to the family room where the student nurse brought them their tea.

In recalling the events that had occurred before Nick's death, Olga regained most of her composure. She relaxed in Maria's comforting presence. There was something about returning to Dunira Hospice. Olga's pain remained, but it was as if the pain hurt less.

Olga told Maria, "In this room I feel safe. For two months I lived here with Nick. And in this family room Nick never felt alone."

Maria, the matriarch of Dunira's extended family, a title bestowed on her by Brian, continued to comfort Olga. Maria exemplified the greatest human qualities of unconditional love and compassion for others.

It is common for palliative care patients, families, and caregivers to reach out to one another. With awareness and humility they understand suffering and in collaboration they form a unique and cohesive self-help group. In her time of need, Olga found Maria's presence a source of comfort and support. At its heart, palliation is all about community and caring for one another.

———

Nick and Olga were born in Ukraine. They immigrated to Canada as postgraduate students and accomplished artists. Canada offered them freedom of choice and freedom of movement. In Canada they found challenges and adventures. The solemnization of their Canadian citizenship had confirmed their allegiance to their new country.

When Nick lost his health and was admitted to Dunira, Olga devoted herself to his care. She seldom left his side. Nick drew comfort from the presence of his wife, who understood his needs. Occasionally, Olga slept in the family room, but mostly she curled up in the big reclining chair beside Nick's bed. Nick was content in the knowledge that Olga would escort him on his last journey home, where he would be buried in the land of his birth. Nick had died peacefully in Olga's arms. With sadness, Olga prepared for his burial and the journey ahead.

———

The reaction of Stan Memorial to Jean's investigative phone call was swift.

The social worker held the funeral home responsible for their callous handling of Olga's call, the way their receptionist had brushed Olga off, and, instead of properly checking, had reported instead the shocking news of the apparent loss of Nick's remains. The social worker emphasized the unnecessary and very real grief caused to Nick's widow by the funeral home's lax and unprofessional behavior.

In response, Stan Memorial set in motion a rush of events. Three-and-a-half hours after Jean's initial phone call, followed by an additional seven phone calls back and forth, a special delivery was arranged. A young man presented himself at Dunira's nursing station. Mr. Youngman requested a meeting with the social worker. Without a moment to lose, Jean appeared on the scene and escorted Mr. Youngman to her office.

From a heavy black bag that he placed on Jean's desk, Mr. Youngman extracted the urn containing Nick's ashes. He then extracted a letter of apology addressed personally to Olga. Before removing the remaining contents from his mysterious black bag, Mr. Youngman discussed his offer to escort Olga home. He further proposed that Stan Memorial provide a cab to take Olga to the airport the day of her departure. Moreover, Mr. Youngman promised to assist Olga with the required regulations concerning her flight and that of her husband's ashes.

Finally, Mr. Youngman handed Jean three large boxes of chocolates.

Jean left Mr. Youngman sitting in her office and went in search of Olga.

Olga graciously accepted the apology of Stan Memorial and thankfully accepted their assistance with the airport protocol regarding her flight to Ukraine. In the company of Mr. Youngman, Olga made a dignified exit home.

It is doubtful that Olga will ever forget the shock that Stan Memorial had caused her. And Jean, the social worker, had let it be known that she would never forget the funeral home's callous disregard of a grieving widow by claiming that they had misplaced Nick's remains simply because they were too busy to stop what they were doing to help her.

Jean deposited the three boxes of chocolates in the conference room, naming them Day, Evening, and Night, compliments of Stan Memorial.

On returning to her office to write her notes on the events of the day, Jean heard Brian's voice as he called out his good-bye. And in listening, she heard Brian say, "Bye you guys. Have a silly day."

As the door closed softly behind him, Jean wondered how Brian had known that indeed they were all in need of a silly day. Jean recalled the fact of seventeen good-byes in one month. And the weight of all those good-byes was daunting.

Four days later, Olga was once again reunited with her motherland. And in death, Nick returned to the place of his birth to be buried by his family.

Mount Pleasant

*The presence of grief must be acknowledged
for as painful as grief may be,
grieving prepares the bereaved for the changes ahead.*

Sharing information with health care practitioners and the public at large was a component of Dunira's palliative mandate. And true to its mandate, Dunira Hospice offered information and discussions on pain management, the alleviation of suffering, family support, and home care services.

Mount Pleasant, a rehab hospital, enjoyed an excellent reputation. Given this reputation for excellence, one wondered what Dunira's palliative care could offer the rehab hospital. Yet a request for palliative intervention had been sought. Before Dunira's staff could reply though, it was necessary to understand the nature of patient care offered at the Mount Pleasant Rehabilitation Hospital.

In sifting through the layers of Mount Pleasant's policy, some disturbing facts came to light. Most patients at the rehab hospital were long-term stay and wheelchair-bound. Professional staff worked towards restoring mobility and body function. Death at the rehab hospital was the exception rather than the rule. Yet during a period of four months, seven young patients had died. The causes of their deaths were not described. What *was* known was the denial of death's presence by rehab staff.

Invariably, death and rehabilitation are diametrically opposed. Death's occurrence within the rehab hospital was regarded as a failure to cure. And the staff grieved in silence. The hospital director believed that a seminar on grief would improve staff morale and enable them to cope with the clinically depressed patients who also mourned the recent deaths.

Death Denial

Upon reflection, the expectations of the hospital's director were unrealistic. To believe that a seminar on grief would eradicate existing problems at the rehab hospital was simplistic. However, in consideration of the patients at Mount Pleasant, Dunira's palliative care team proposed that Head Nurse Claire and Sister Beatrice offer a discussion on the subject of grief and loss.

It came to light that hospital policy at Mount Pleasant stipulated full bed occupancy. All vacated, sanitized beds were in such demand that they were immediately occupied by new and waiting patients. Bound by the terms of hospital policy, staff was obliged to act with haste and strip away all traces of former patient occupants.

But to proceed without ceremony, to remove all traces of a deceased person, then offer the vacated bed to a new and waiting patient is an act of profanity. For such an act tries to negate the presence of death and disregards death's impact on both patients and staff.

Conspiracy of Silence

The staff at Mount Pleasant had unwittingly caused suffering for their patients when in silent haste they removed all traces of the deceased patients.

In addition, their silence served to fan the flames of fear.

In four short months, seven patients had died at the rehab hospital. Yet staff had remained mute, as if death had not occurred. A simple memorial service to commemorate the dead and acknowledge the presence of grief would have supported both vulnerable patients and hospital staff. But there were no memorial services and the latent manifestations of such an oversight had a negative impact on patients and staff alike. As a result, an atmosphere of tension, of silence without meaning, hung like a dark oppressive cloud over Mount Pleasant.

Where was the humanity in this?

Oppressive silence caused mourning and filled the air with desolate despair. Those with wheels instead of legs had many questions left unasked.

Seven friends had been there, seven friends who had burned with fierce humanity. Yet they had vanished without a trace. Were they merely phantoms passing through?

Grief and Loss

When a relationship ends in death, we need time to mourn. We need time to find our way through life's complex maze. Social rituals enable us to express joy and sadness when, for instance, we celebrate birth or mourn death. Rituals such as the funeral, the wake, and the memorial service confirm that death has occurred and allow us to honor the dead. Social rituals enable us to frame our lives.

Yet sadly, in our English-speaking culture, death is taboo.

Death is ambiguous for it is cloaked in a tattered shroud of mystery and secrecy. Is it any wonder that we fear death yet remain preoccupied with dying?

We are guided through the steps of burial by the funeral director. Yet in providing this vital service to humanity, the funeral director perpetuates the mystery surrounding death.

I once asked a funeral director, "How do you attend to the expression of grief? How do you support the bereaved?"

In response the funeral director replied, "I become very matter-of-fact. I become very businesslike."

To which I responded, "In other words, you disallow and discourage the expression of grief."

And yet the visible presence of grief must be acknowledged. For painful and grim as grief may be, grieving prepares the bereaved for the changes they must face, changes that lie ahead.

On the day of the grief seminar, Head Nurse Claire and Sister Beatrice met with the director of Mount Pleasant Hospital. They were welcomed with distant formality and politely escorted to the hospital auditorium, where the proposed discussion on grief and loss was to be conducted.

Claire and Beatrice were astounded by the awesome scene of the hospital auditorium. A podium resembling a pulpit stood in front of an endless sea of chairs, where several staff members sat in anticipation of a lecture on grief and loss. But such a lecture would be meaningless. For grief is not a sickness of the mind to be eradicated in ten or fifteen easy steps. Grief is similar to anguish of the soul because of damage to the self.

Little did staff know that the women from Dunira had come to help staff express themselves about life's ending. Both Claire and Beatrice had prepared themselves to facilitate an exchange of unrestrained communication about the denial of death's presence and its impact on our lives.

Claire and Beatrice aimed to create a process of healing, enabling patients and staff to interact with one another and acknowledge grief's presence in death's wake. The women planned to offer themselves to patients and staff as willing companions in a meaningful exchange of communication about a subject that creates undisclosed pain.

Breaking through Silence

A young man wheeled his way towards Claire, the head nurse. A brace immobilized his head. But the quiet sound of his rolling wheels was like thunder to Claire's ears, for he had roused her from a reverie. Claire witnessed the pain reflected in his eyes. She told the young man, "I need you here. I hope you'll stay. We must lift this veil of silence that has caused such distress."

One by one the patients came and quietly remained.

Sister Beatrice clapped her hands, as was her usual way, and in a most persuasive voice she said, "Claire and I are here to give ourselves away to each and every one of you. And in turn you will also give yourselves away. But before we receive your gifts, let's rearrange this room. We'll make a circle that's loose enough to accommodate wheelchairs and tight enough to make a caring chain of communication."

With haste they rearranged that awesome, sterile room.

Light poured in and light remained.

Sister Beatrice's voice rang out. "Before we can begin, I'll tell you the story of a charming young man. The young man in my story is blind."

Gathered in a circle, patients and rehab staff listened to the story of the courageous blind man:

He was a proud young man
And thinking to retain his dignity,
And his independence, and cover up his loss of sight,
He walked along the busy streets,
No seeing-eye dog to guide him,
No symbolic white cane.
He walked on, listening to the heavy traffic on the road.
Courageous and determined he prevailed.
Until one day his hearing ears did not detect
The bicycle following from behind
Until too late!
The soundless bicycle knocked the young man down.

The story told by Sister Beatrice opened a tide of conversation.

The communication flowed like a river that burst its banks, washing away silent, unseen obstacles and boundaries. Every man and every woman present in that chain of communication found meaning in the story of the proud blind man.

Rituals Enable Us to Frame Our Lives

Someone in the group said, "Society once had the means to identify the bereaved. Men wore black armbands and women wore black 'widow's weeds.'"

The apparel of those in grief once identified them in their time of mourning and made each of us aware of their need for consideration and care. Yes, ceremonial rituals are of great significance in our lives.

In response, Head Nurse Claire said, "Nature leads the way in honor of birth and death. Just look around at the changing seasons. The seasons give meaning to the passage of time and frame the events in our lives."

And in that circle of communication, that human chain, the participants opened up. They gave themselves to one another and chased away their fears. With brave, bold strokes they breathed life into the portraits of seven absent friends. Memories to cherish gave way to smiles and tears. Each person acknowledged that in grief's sore, gnawing pain there is meaning, and meaning brings relief.

What happened in that circle was memorable, heart-warming, and useful. A new ritual had been created for the Mount Pleasant community.

Social rituals enrich and enable us to frame our lives.

Even more than that, in unison the participants broke the conspiracy of silence that surrounded seven absent friends. Memories to treasure were etched upon their minds. They were no longer plagued by fear of phantom ghosts, because they had chased those ghosts away.

Someone in the group asked both Claire and Beatrice, "Will you come again?"

And with humility, both women answered, "Yes."

What had the Dunira's palliative care team offered the staff and patients at Mount Pleasant Rehabilitation Hospital?

Palliative care had offered a way for the staff and the patients to lift the veil of silence from their grief and to acknowledge the value and meaning of life and the patient/caregiver relationship.

Through the Camera Lens: Emma

One fleeting moment frozen by the camera, what image do you see?
Does it reveal your bias?
Does it blind you to the vibrant colors of the fabric
that shape a person's life?

A local broadcasting company was given permission by the administration at the Acute Care Hospital to make a documentary about Dunira Hospice. Dr. Daniel did not approve of the administration's decision because he believed that the presence of a television crew in the Hospice was inappropriate. Despite his protest, he was unable to halt the process.

While the proposed documentary about palliative care might prove its worth in educational value, the reality of such a venture was disruptive.

Dr. Daniel expressed his frustration to Claire, the head nurse. "What do they hope to achieve by making a documentary of Dunira? How can you capture the essence of palliative care with a camera? They just don't know that it's only when you wipe a patient's bum and clear away the vomit that you begin to understand what it's all about. Understanding comes with doing, when you grasp the nettle and get on with whatever needs to be done."

Hospice is a place for critically ill patients who require a safe, noninvasive environment. Preserving the sensitivity of the palliative care environment was paramount. Dr. Daniel demanded the assurance of the television crew that the making of the documentary would not place patient care in jeopardy.

The administration agreed that the proposed documentary might impede the daily routine at Dunira, but insisted that the educational value of the documentary for the public would outweigh any inconvenience incurred.

But oh, the cost of that education once Alec Smart launched himself on the scene. His version of the world was captured through a narrow camera lens. Restricted by his bias, the television producer sought the lengthening shadows, the dark within the light. Without caution, sensitivity, or humility, Alec Smart proceeded with his documentary. He allowed nothing to delay his deadline. But as Mr. Smart went about his task, he invited Emma's rage and extinguished Emma's light.

And so it was that the world of Emma, a seriously ill patient, collided with the world of a stranger, a television man by the name of Alec Smart.

Skilled in the craft of manipulation, Alec Smart expected patients to comply with his needs. In the manner of an authoritarian, he showed a lack of consideration for those he interviewed. And as if it was his right, he accosted Emma with the demand, "Let me be your confidant. Help me understand what it's like to die. The answers you give will help others understand."

What Mr. Smart failed to understand was the audacity of his request.

Dying is profound, unique, and deeply personal. For enshrined therein is the essence of our being, our body, mind and soul.

Emma was rightly affronted and lost control. Her emergency light summoned the head nurse. Claire arrived to find Emma ashen white and deeply distressed.

"Who is that hotshot TV Man?" Emma asked. "What gives him the right to come in here? I don't care about his documentary. I don't want him near me again. Claire, sort him out! He can't come in here and trample all over us."

The making of the documentary had placed Emma in jeopardy. She should not have been subjected to the intrusive assault of Alec Smart's interrogation. Mr. Smart lacked diplomacy and had discounted his responsibility to tread softly. Without question, the ultimate responsibility for the safety and comfort of the patients at Dunira fell squarely on the shoulders of hospice staff.

Claire's response to Emma's plea was immediate. She went in search of the television man and found him in the conference room.

Full of indignation, Mr. Smart complained, "Your patients won't talk to me. I had high hopes for that little gal 'cross the hall. But she's a real hothead. Can't imagine why she got so mad. Never mind. Tomorrow there'll be staff interviews. Might get lucky. Make some progress."

Claire closed the door of the conference room and in a voice of deadly calm said, "Sir, have you forgotten that you are a guest at Dunira? As for making progress—progress will be made if you mind how you go! Mr. Smart, please know that we do not hang crepes here. We do not bury people before they are dead."

The head nurse continued, "It's all quite simple really. But first, put your own agenda aside. Have some compassion and open your ears to really hear. And in listening, invite our patients to share a chapter from their *Book of Life*. Then stand aside. Our patients will decide whether they wish to share with you some highlight of their journey, some aspect of their life's adventure. Talk to our patients about the challenge of living life."

Claire paused for a moment then told the television man, "Sir, you need to understand that at Dunira, we work as a team. We take our directions from our patients and their families."

Alec Smart was stunned into silence.

But he heard Claire's words as she reproached him, "It was my understanding that your interests lay in the provision of care to patients and families at Dunira. Never for one moment did I think your documentary represented the physical dramatization of death."

As the head nurse walked away, she knew that Alec Smart's complaints were directed not only at those patients who rejected the drama of his script, his complaints were directed at her. Alec Smart did not want to be told what to do and he objected to Claire's interference.

Alec Smart ignored the delicate balance between hope and despair. He did not understand that a lack of optimistic or positive interaction with terminally ill patients is likely to contribute to their sense of helplessness. He was a stranger who boldly demanded that Emma reveal her private self. Without awareness or sensitivity, he had interrogated her as if it was his right. And she, vulnerable and fragile, had responded with justifiable outrage to his prodding. Emma's anger preserved her rights and defended her dignity as a person.

Anticipation of the termination of one's life is an awesome process and comprehension of such a process is formidable. The dying person assumes the role of a patient and, in so doing, surrenders much of their independence to caregivers.

Emma disliked being a patient and she hated to talk about her illness. Although she was seriously ill, Emma had not lost her capacity for the bliss of life. Indeed, she appeared to cling to all that was good.

A Pristine Wintry Scene

After a restless night of rumination and troubled dreams, Head Nurse Claire stood in awe of the early morning. Layers of crunchy, glistening snow covered the ground and gently hushed the waking city. A heavy frost had visited the elm and willow trees, and their branches shimmered in a mantle of delicate lace. The wide-open sky welcomed another precious day. And as she pondered the unfolding of her day, Claire found relief in the stillness and the beauty of the wintry scene.

When Claire arrived at Dunira, the night nurse's report was in progress. Head Nurse Claire was greeted with the news that Emma had spent a poor night and had lapsed into an unconscious state at 0400 hours. In appearance, Emma resembled a tiny wax doll. Her raven-black hair was brushed and held in place with a tortoise comb. The rich, deep color of Emma's hair contrasted sharply with the pallor of her skin.

Mavis, another hospice patient, shared a room with Emma. And with the passion of one who is protecting her friend, Mavis told Claire, "Emma looks like she's suspended somewhere. She was waiting for Hugh. And him coming all the way from Alaska to see his mum. I guess Emma just couldn't hold on."

Mavis burst into tears. "I hate to go home and leave Emma like this. How can I go home without saying good-bye? Everybody's so sick in here. It was an awful thought to come here, especially since my family promised me that I could stay home. But my doctor told me that they needed a break. And I know he was right."

Mavis paused for a moment, then told Claire, "There's one thing I know for sure. It was Emma who gave me a shot in the arm. She kept on telling me to smile. Don't look so glum 'cause we're still above ground. Emma told me about *The Precious Present*. Some book she'd read. '*We have to make the most out of every single moment.*' That's what she said. She made me laugh."

Mavis spoke about the television crew. Then added, "Emma has nicknames for everybody. She was so feisty with that TV man. The Inquisitor, she calls him. She loves Dr. Daniel, calls him The Saint. And Claire, she calls you Scottie. Marty is our favorite night nurse. Emma calls her Old Bossy Boots. Emma loves to argue with Marty and nearly always wins. But Marty is so good. She just laughs and brings us a glass of sherry."

Claire reflected on the relationship that had developed between Emma and Mavis and noted that they were quietly at peace. This reflection led the head nurse to suggest to Mavis: "In the quietness of the evening, talk to Emma. She can't answer you, but she'll hear your voice. And Mavis, she needs to hear your voice. Tell Emma about all your precious moments. And ask Old Bossy Boots to sing Emma a song. Ask her to sing 'Ain't Misbehavin'.' That song always made Emma laugh."

Miracles Sometimes Happen

Emma remained comatose for more than thirty-six hours. Could it be that in order to conserve her dwindling energy

Emma had removed herself from the unusual hustle and bustle of the television crew?

Now in limbo, out of touch, out of reach, and disconnected, Emma remained in a protective cocoon. Barely alive, she was waiting for her son. Emma had waited a long time for this final visit with her son. She knew that time was not on her side. But there were things to be done. There were urgent things that Emma needed to tell Hugh, her only son.

During the time she remained unconscious, Emma's nurses tended to her, bathed her, and gently massaged her back and limbs to prevent the occurrence of sore pressure points. The nurses turned her every two hours and a slow intravenous saline solution kept Emma hydrated. Her roommate, Mavis, and the nurses took it in turn to keep Emma's lips and mouth moist. During that period of uncertainty, Mavis kept vigil. And Dr. Daniel visited and marked up Emma's calendar. Hospice volunteers took it in turn to sit with Emma. They gently stroked her fingers, thereby maintaining the life-sustaining communication of touch.

Was the miracle of Emma's making? Of that, no one can be sure. It is enough to say that she willed herself to stay alive.

Emma caused a wonderful distraction on the unit when she roused herself from her deep slumber and in a voice barely audible, a voice as thin as tissue paper, asked the nurses in her room, "Where have you been?"

Head Nurse Claire teased back. "Oh, away with you, Emma. You're such a wee blether. We've been here all the time. But where have *you* been? Where have *you* been hiding?"

"I went to the other side," Emma whispered. "But they weren't ready for me. So I'm back." Then she asked, "Is Mavis here? And what about Hugh? Is Hugh here?"

Emma's nurse picked up the calendar, then she bent close to Emma's ear and said, "Look at this. Dr. Daniel marked your calendar. Your son arrives tonight. And as for Mavis, she is right here. She's been waiting for you to wake up."

Mavis found her voice and said, "No doubt about it, Emma, Old Bossy Boots'll be serving us sherry tonight."

"There's time for several naps before Hugh arrives," Claire told Emma. Then she added in a firm voice, "But no hiding too far away, okay? And just so you know, Emma, we'll be in and out to keep an eye on you."

Emma's son, Hugh, arrived late in the afternoon that very same day. And for the briefest time, just long enough to sort his mother's affairs, Emma regained her sparkle and looked as if she had recovered her health. But it was not another miracle. It was simply that Emma had mustered all her life forces, her energy, and her courage to make the last four days of her life memorable for herself and her son.

It was time for Mavis to go home. Her family arrived and she said farewell to Emma and her son. Mavis was happy to be going home, yet saddened to say good-bye to Emma.

Hugh remained with his mother, wanting to spend their last precious moments together. And just as Olga and many other family members had done, Hugh slept in Dunira's family room. But the night before his mother died, Hugh stayed in the big reclining chair at his mother's bedside.

Emma was content in the knowledge that everything now lay in the capable hands of her son. And, after the whisper of a gentle sigh, she died.

Lives in Progress

The palliative care team labored with tireless hands and feet to make the transition from hospice a comfortable passage for Paul's weekend pass home. And, in turn, the nurses welcomed Vladimir and supported his wife, whose grief was so hard to bear.

Vladie's Gift of Sharing

Vladie was admitted to Dunira for respite care. His readmission to the hospice was a matter of coming and going for the reassessment of his pain. And when he left, he took with him a new pain regimen.

But Vladie was never really free from pain. Once he told Head Nurse Claire, "You mustn't try to take away all my pain because my pain tells me where my cancer's taking me."

Vladie loved to tell his stories of the Old Country and his happy days as a student engineer in Portugal. When Vladie moved into his stories, his pain lost some of its sharp edges. And in recounting the tales of long ago, he became more relaxed and enjoyed a restful sleep.

More than once Vladie told Claire, "When you get to Heaven, you'll know a lot of people up there."

Vladie wanted Claire to know that death was more friend than foe. Vladie no longer feared death's presence.

To share Vladie's intimate thoughts of his impending death made Claire a privileged listener. They talked about important things that needed to be said.

And in telling her, "You mustn't try to take away all my pain," Vladie expressed his trust and regard.

The reciprocal relationship that exists between patients and palliative caregivers was maintained. The marvel of such relationships in palliative care is secured by giving and receiving within a community of support, where we find ways to make things better than they are.

Jessie's Independence

Words were always at hand when Jessie needed them. So much so that she never left anyone in doubt as to what was on her mind. And there was a lot on Jessie's mind.

Her daughter, Myra, and son, Ronald, had almost convinced Jessie that her admission to Dunira Hospice was urgent. Jessie's pain was within manageable limits, thanks to the skill of her family doctor. Jessie herself struggled to manage persistent fatigue, but frequent catnaps sustained her.

So why did her family make such a fuss? Surely they knew that home was the only place that Jessie wanted to be.

But Jessie's words of protest, even her words of wisdom, fell on the deaf ears of her son and her daughter. They discounted home as an option for Jessie because the doctor's diagnosis and his referral for their mother's admission to Dunira rang loudly in their ears. But in spite of the doctor's diagnosis, and regardless of her uncertain health, Jessie told her family she was capable of making her own decisions. She intended to remain at home. Worn down by the back and forth persuasion of her family, and in a state of pessimistic defeat, Jessie finally agreed to be admitted to Dunira Hospice.

Swathed in her Harris tweed suit, now three sizes too large, and dwarfed in a pea-green hat, a disconsolate Jessie arrived at Dunira in the company of her family. Having comfortably settled her mother, Myra presented herself at the open door of the social worker. Jean seldom closed her office door because she knew that family members often had a need to talk about their present and uncertain futures.

MOTHER IS UNSINKABLE

Myra talked to Jean about her mother.

"Why didn't I realize that mother was so ill? She was always independent. That's how she was. That's how it was all her life. I never guessed she was ill. She only recently stopped driving around delivering Meals on Wheels. Last year she went out and bought a house on the edge of town and never even mentioned it until the deed was done!"

Myra continued as if giving voice to her worries. "I hope she won't be a problem here. She didn't want to come!"

Jean listened to Myra's concerns.

"Mother is like the Unsinkable Molly Brown," Myra added with a sigh. "Will you call me at the first sign of any difficulties with her?"

The social worker assured Myra that she and her brother

would be kept informed of their mother's progress. Moreover, both would be invited to participate in Jessie's plan of care.

Jean continued, "Family participation is an expectation at Dunira." Then she held out her hand to Myra, smiled, and said, "Let's go and see your mother. I'd like to meet the Unsinkable Molly Brown."

Jessie acknowledged the social worker's presence, then looking Jean straight in the eye silently begged to be rescued.

From that first encounter, Jessie had it figured that somehow the social worker would be an ally in her bid for freedom.

During those early days at Dunira, Jessie was a model patient. But Dr. Daniel was not deceived by her quiet demeanor. Jessie's mind, as always, was fully occupied making secret plans for discharge.

Grudgingly, Jessie admitted feeling less tired, but added, "This place does nothing to improve my mood."

Jessie had been at Dunira for less than a week when she made her move and showed her hand. She told the dietitian, "I could kill for a fresh carrot muffin and a soft-boiled egg."

Jessie then turned her attention to the social worker. "Sit here beside me. I need to talk to you. Tell me, how did you get a job like this? I mean all you ever do is talk to people. Still I suppose there's something to be said for talking. I could do your job. I'm just like you. And I love to talk. Do you need any special training for your job?"

In response to Jessie's inquiry, Jean asked, "Jessie, something is bothering you. Can you tell me what's on your mind?"

"I hate this place," Jessie said. "Mind you I think it's fine for some people. But everybody's dying here. And some of them don't even have friends. I want to go home. But my family won't hear of it. They think that I don't know what's wrong with me. We play such ridiculous games my kids and me. We pretend everything's fine. But my Rab knows. He understands. I talk to Rab all the time. He helps me figure things out. He was such a good husband. Brave as could be. My Rab was a fireman. He died saving a child from a horrible blaze. Looking back, I don't think I've been a good mother 'cause I always put Rab first. Mind you, our kids never wanted for anything and their friends were always welcome in our home."

Jessie paused as if trying to read Jean's mind before continuing. "My friends are widows just like me. All our husbands were firemen. When we were young we stuck together because we never knew when trouble would come. That's how it was. And over the years we kept in touch."

Jessie waited another moment. "When my Rab died, my friends pulled me through. I don't know what I would have done without them. I have four good friends and we do things together. We play whist every Wednesday. And we have a potluck supper on Fridays. When I go home, my friends will help me. Of course, I might just drop dead. What if I just dropped dead?"

Jean, the social worker, replied, "My dear wise Jessie, is that what you want? To be at home with caring friends who are close to you?"

"Yes," Jessie said without hesitation. "Yes. Above all else, I want to go home. Will you help me? Please?"

Much to Jessie's delight, the social worker replied, "Don't worry about your family's reluctance to your going home. I've got a card up my sleeve. All will be well."

Along the way, Jessie had used others as a yardstick to measure her own failing health. She knew that she was dying, and when she caught a glimpse of herself in the mirror, she responded with humor. Her daughter would say in haste, "Now don't be alarmed, Mother. I always knew there was something wrong with that mirror."

But for Jessie all that really mattered was to live and die at home. There was much to be done. So Jean, the social worker, Head Nurse Claire, and Dr. Daniel put their heads together and arranged a preliminary family meeting for Jessie.

On the day of Jessie's family meeting at Dunira, the hospice volunteer placed a pot of coffee, six mugs, cream, and sugar on the conference room table. The coffee was a warm welcome for Jessie's family. And Dr. Daniel's gracious presence encouraged Myra and her brother, Ronald, to be at ease. Then the meeting got underway.

Myra and Ronald asked many questions of the small informal group gathered around the conference table.

Dr. Daniel said, "We are not here to dissuade your mother from her wish to go home. Our coming together like this will help us find answers and solutions that will work. And together we will plan your mother's care. Jessie has shared her point of view with us and we want to meet her needs. We understood her when she said that being at Dunira didn't fit the bill. You know, it's not a bad idea to live and die at home. And without a doubt, your mother wants to live and die at home."

Myra asked, "But how will she be able to manage at home alone?"

Jean, the social worker, told Myra, "Your mother won't be at home alone. That's why we're here. To plan the services she'll need."

Head Nurse Claire also sought to reassure Myra. "This first meeting is a way of identifying the services your mother will need. Once we know what's needed, we'll work together to sort things out. Then we'll put everything in place."

Ronald, who up to that point had not spoken, suddenly found his voice. "I'm opposed to my mother's discharge."

Dr. Daniel gently confirmed that Dunira would not keep a patient against her will. Then he reminded Ronald and Myra, "Your mother has an independent spirit. And that is something we value at Dunira. Jessie is relatively free of pain on her current medications. Her medications will be continued. And I will contact her family doctor to inform him of her discharge plan. Your mother is independently mobile. She has a clear, sharp mind. And with a plan of care firmly in place, she should be comfortable and safe."

Ronald asked, "How much time does Mother have?"

In reply, Dr. Daniel said, "No one can predict when a person will die. Using statistical information to inform a patient or a family of the time of death is at best an educated guess. And that's not a guess we practice at Dunira."

In spite of reassurance for his mother's continued care, Ronald told the group, "I'm unhappy to think of Mother going home."

The social worker asked Ronald, "Is it really in your mother's best interest to remain at Dunira?"

Ronald didn't respond.

Jean played her ace, that one card up her sleeve. Her voice rang out as she said, "Your mother may choose to discharge herself. It's entirely within her rights. Although she's ill, she's of sound mind. Her intentions and decisions must be honored. Besides, Jessie has enough cash on hand to hire a cab and take herself home. And if she were my mother, I wouldn't want her to go home alone."

Head Nurse Claire added, "We must accept Jessie's wishes and attempt to meet her needs. We must cooperate with one another. Jessie trusts us to provide her home care and that's what's important here."

The back and forth discussion between the family and the palliative team, the questions asked and answered, helped resolve the fear of Myra and Ronald that their mother would indeed receive the professional care she needed at home. And they came to accept that their mother had rights that needed to be respected.

At the conclusion of the meeting, Dr. Daniel said, "It's essential that we attempt to understand how Jessie views her world. For that is more important than how anyone of us feels. Your mother has cooperated with everyone on Dunira's team. We must also cooperate with her."

Finally, with the agreement of Jessie's family, a new discharge meeting was arranged, one that Jessie would attend.

Prior to the planned discharge meeting, Jessie's family doctor was informed of her requirements for palliative home care. The doctor responded by confirming that both palliative nursing and homemaker services would be securely in place.

Jessie's team of family and four friends met with Dr. Daniel, Head Nurse Claire, and Jean, the social worker. In Jessie's presence, and with her agreement, her discharge plan was put in place.

The plan was similar to a written contract of commitment. Jessie's friends agreed to take turns staying overnight. And, in effect, Jessie's care plan became a duty roster that covered a twenty-four-hour day.

One of Jessie's friends shared her thoughts. "It'll be like the old days. When we stood together and faced what needed to be done."

At last the conflict was resolved. Jessie was going home.

From her wheelchair carriage, Jessie bade us farewell. She was going on a journey to her special place at home. Wrapped in her old, warm tweeds and looking out from under that green felt hat, Jessie sat serene.

Yes indeed, Jessie was in the driver's seat.

Jessie knew our hospice arms were long and that our long arms stretched out into the community. And if needed, we would not hesitate to reach her.

POINSETTIAS IN PROFUSION

The windowsill of every available window ledge at Dunira Hospice held vases of fragrant flowers. Clay pots and wicker baskets were filled with red and white poinsettias. The poinsettias were a gift from Jessie's family. And those Christmas blooms reminded everyone of Jessie and her spirit of fire.

Wednesday was the day of Jessie's favorite card game. Her friends gathered round the kitchen table at her home for their weekly game of whist. But soon Jessie tired.

Unable to finish the game, she told her friends, "I need a nap."

Early evening approached when Jessie's friends tiptoed into her room to rouse her for tea. Jessie lay in bed as if asleep. But Jessie, lying quiet and still, had passed away in peace. Jessie had died in her sleep.

Thanks to the care of her family and friends, Jessie lived and died in the comfort of her home, living every moment in the "*precious present*".

Jessie's family and friends had dipped deep into their reserves and discovered a source of strength that empowered them, giving meaning and purpose to their interdependent relationships and selfless compassion.

A Forum for Palliative Care

Death is ambiguous
for it is cloaked in a shroud of mystery and secrecy.
Is it any wonder that we fear death yet remain preoccupied with dying?

Conferences provide a forum for experts and international speakers to share their expertise on a variety of topics central to the provision of palliative care. International palliative care conferences are hosted in cities throughout the world. An important aspect of bringing people together to confer is to fulfill the need for providers and consumers to understand what palliative medicine offers to the quality of care for the terminally ill.

One such conference comprised a group of approximately a hundred people, including providers and consumers of hospice care, who had come together to discuss palliative care. Sister Beatrice, Head Nurse Claire, and two hospice volunteers from Dunira were also in attendance.

The program of events indicated that a staff member from Dunira Hospice would introduce a documentary film on palliative care.

When Head Nurse Claire agreed to introduce Alec Smart's documentary, she assumed that she and Sister Beatrice would simply answer questions about palliative patient care services at Dunira Hospice and within the community. But foolishly, neither woman had viewed the documentary prior to its introduction at the conference. And both regretted their error.

They assumed that Alec Smart's documentary portrayed the quality of compassionate hospice patient care. Unbeknownst to Claire and Beatrice, Smart's film was biased toward the drama of life's termination; it was a film that portrayed a lopsided view of life and living, of death and dying.

Alec Smart's film betrayed the very essence and flavor of Dunira. There was no laughter, no music, no whispering songsters in Brian's longhouse. No mention of the wedding of Grace and Gordon. The marvelous seafaring stories of Jock and the sea captain were absent from the documentary. The viewing audience did not see the joy on Emma's face as she listened to her son's stories of adventures in Alaska. There was no hint of Dunira's many celebrations, birthdays, anniversaries, and achievements.

The viewing audience was unaware of Dunira's unique self-help group, comprised of those extended family members who offered assistance and support to needy others. Moreover, the documentary failed to provide information about the ongoing support group for families.

Instead, the film focused on one dying man and placed him under a microscope as if to examine the physical occurrence of death.

Head Nurse Claire was disarmed by the empty gloom of Smart's documentary. In Claire's view, those who had made the film and those who viewed the film remained spectators, outsiders, no wiser than before. To Claire, the film distorted reality because it did nothing to convey the essence of humanity and compassion in the art of palliative care.

Palliative care may be likened to the parable of the Good Samaritan who offered compassion and nonjudgmental care to a fellow traveler along the way. Palliative caring is a special branch of medicine that offers comfort care to patients and their families. When a cure is no longer possible, palliative care seeks to alleviate suffering in an environment of support, dignity, and respect.

Following the presentation of the misleading documentary, Claire found herself in the center of a group of pastoral care and lay participants. With unabated curiosity, the group sought answers to the unanswerable. And all of them asked many questions of Claire.

One persistent voice asked Claire, "How did you get into this work?"

"I have no instant answer to your question," Claire replied. "But given my poor sense of direction, it may well be that my work found me."

Someone else asked, "What are you? Are you a nurse or a social worker?"

"I am a nurse and social worker, wife, mother, aunt, friend, and grandmother."

Questions unrelated to palliative care followed in quick succession:

"Are you deeply religious?"

"Do you believe in God?"

"How do you handle stress?"

"Does your family support you in your work?"

"Do you fear death? Or is death just commonplace to you?"

Claire's answers to the many questions asked of her failed to satisfy the group. No answer that she might offer could satisfy their avid curiosity, because they remained outside the situation. They were spectators, curious observers of life and living, and of death and dying.

Dissatisfied, the group dispersed, leaving Claire alone with many questions of her own. Claire wondered why there was such a need to focus on the physical process of dying. After all, dying is less than a fraction of a moment in the life of any person.

Is not the life of a person the more important aspect of our living experience?

Claire disliked Alec Smart's docudrama. It left her restless and ill at ease.

What an intrusion! Where was the dignity for the patient? Mr. Roland's last living moments were captured through the lens of a camera and showed nothing of his humanity, nothing of his gentle presence, nothing of his reality or that of his ailing, aged wife.

Alec Smart had captured Mr. Ronald's noisy, stertorous breathing, often referred to as the "death rattle." Claire felt outraged. She wondered whose needs had been met in the making and the showing of Smart's documentary. What was the purpose of this presentation at a so-called Hospice Palliative Care Conference?

Some might argue that the film was educational and that

was purpose enough. For Claire though, the documentary was nothing more than a dramatization of the physical process of death. Sick at heart, Claire believed that the film served only to reinforce a void between the living and the dying.

Perhaps the real result of Alec Smart's docudrama was nothing more than a perpetuation of our society's fear of death.

Answers to questions of terminal illness and death are ambiguous, perhaps best left to artists and poets, who, with mastery, reveal the enigmas confronting each and every one of us in our journey through life.

Interdependent Relationships: Heather

Illness inflicts suffering on both patients and family.

How sad that in the pursuit of *cure*, health care personnel pay very little attention to the importance of relationships. Yet in the provision of patient *care*, families play a major role. Earlier in this book, we witnessed Sofia's abject despair when hospital staff ignored her concerns and prevented her contribution towards her husband's care.

The importance of the family-patient relationship is well documented. Cecily Saunders recognized the patient-family as the "unit of care."[16] Findings of others, like Balfour Mount and Eric J. Cassell, further confirm that families provide the primary source of emotional support for seriously ill patients. Recognition and acceptance of interdependent relationships between patients, families, and professional caregivers is crucial in caring for the seriously ill and is fundamental to the philosophy of palliative care.

The story of Heather reveals the strength and importance of family relations.

Heather's small upright piano stood untouched in the center of her room. Yet there was a time when music filled her life. By way of explanation she said, "I have collected all my music.

I want to give it away. I'll feel much lighter then. Father must have this album of songs by the great masters. Music changed my life. But I don't need it now."

No need for music? How could that be? Music was her life, as vital as the very act of breathing.

She complained about the cold weather saying, "My body is too thin. I can't chase away this ice-cold chill. It's with me every day. And I dread the snow." Suddenly she fell silent, then lifted her hands up to hold her painful head.

Heather's mother wrapped her love around her daughter, pulling a blanket up to her daughter's chin.

What sense was to be made of what she said? No sense at all. It was her illness speaking, illness that distorted thoughts and burdened her uneasy mind.

Not long before, music had filled her life, snowflakes fell around her, and never did she mind. Winter's chill was furthest thing from her mind when she arranged a sleigh ride on the frozen Bow River. And on that sleigh ride, she led her choir in a joyful chorus of Christmas carols and good cheer. Two Clydesdale horses hitched to the heavy cart were the gentle giants that carried Heather and her songsters across the frozen reaches of the river.

The presence of a malignant tumor inside Heather's head was unknown to anyone at that time. The tumor forced her on a journey along a disconnected path of treacherous dark moods and pain. To acknowledge the presence of a tumor that invades the brain is to face an awful fear of the unknown. It changed Heather's world forever.

But for Heather, the changes just kept coming. After a difficult and traumatic surgery, she was rendered brain-injured and permanently handicapped.

Who could possibly understand the trauma experienced by Heather and her family? Who could understand the suffering during Heather's illness, the unexpected outcome of her surgery, her daily struggles to regain purpose, hope, and ability in the days, months, and years that followed?

The changes caused by illness brought Heather inequality because hospital staff classified her as a non-compliant patient. But Heather refused to become a compliant member of that unfortunate minority of the brain-injured. She deviated from what is considered normal according to the expectations of health care personnel because she fought to regain her personhood, her individuality.

Heather's brain injury resulted in an onslaught of remarks, opinions, and judgments that were negative and entirely without foundation. Heather and her family were showered with insensitive and cruel remarks, such as "Brain tumors are silent and unobtrusive." "They are invisible ships that sail by and escape our notice." "Don't be sad! God has other plans for your daughter." Even, "It must be Hell to be the parents of that girl with the lobotomy."

Remarks like these reveal the absence of compassion and understanding. Undoubtedly, the result of such remarks serves no other purpose than to create a vulnerable and further victimized patient and family.

Suffering Identified

Where are the lifelines for the critically ill
in the aftermath of brain surgery?
Who will understand the enormity of suffering of the injured mind?
Where is meaning to be found?

Oh, what anguish Heather suffered following the surgery on her brain.

And what anguished awareness for her father, who kept vigil for his daughter, as she lay motionless on that hospital bed, unable to speak, unable to move. The chilling sounds that issued from her throat were, in her father's words, "Like the piercing cries of an animal gripped in a deadly trap." All he could think of was that his firstborn child would surely die.

Willing her to stay alive, he softly told her stories of being once again a child, of finding joy in music. And all night long he saw the tears in his daughter's eyes. He talked to her of concerts when she was full-grown, a person first and foremost, and a fine classical musician. And he recalled Heather's extensive repertoire of music from Bach to Shostakovich that she performed at Carnegie Hall. And in his mind he heard her sing his beloved Gaelic songs.

It was almost dawn when Heather, lulled to sleep by her father's voice, found release.

Throughout that endless night in the acute care hospital, nurses monitored Heather's vital signs, her pulse, blood pressure, and respiration. Their silence was unnerving. There were no words of comfort for this father and his daughter. No offer of a family care meeting to offer support.

The person that was Heather had been rendered helpless by the surgery on her brain. She was left paralyzed and unable to speak. Preoccupation with postoperative symptoms dominated her caregivers' time. No steps were taken to relieve the terror of thoughts that swept through Heather's mind. No small acts of compassion were offered. No touch of a hand, no kind or comforting words. Without her family's support, Heather would have been completely isolated and left alone with her fears.

In *The New England Journal of Medicine*, Dr. E. J. Cassell states that:

> "The question of suffering and its relation to organic illness has rarely been addressed in medical literature. . . . Suffering is experienced by persons, not merely by bodies, and has its source in challenges that threaten the intactness of the person as a complex social and psychological entity."[17]

Heather's stay in the acute care hospital was punitive and long. In that hospital she was identified *only* as a patient, *only* as a set of symptoms. But she refused to accept that role. The caregivers negated Heather's identity and social standing within society. And Heather raged against this negativism of the patient role that deprived her of her personhood.

Surgical Injury of the Brain

The surgery on Heather's brain had impaired her speech and left her paralyzed.

Heather struggled to express her thoughts, but those thoughts were misunderstood. Her slow, painful speech discouraged communication and created boundaries of misunderstanding.

As a result, lifeline therapists focused exclusively on Heather's body and speech. They provided physiotherapy, occupational therapy, speech therapy with instructions that directed her "to accept the loss of her mobility and forge a link between other brain-injured people and herself."

Yet if Heather had merely broken a leg, would they have suggested she forge a link with others with broken legs?

Heather refused the role of helpless patient. Through courage and determination, she fought to retain her individuality as a living, thinking person.

But Heather's nonconformity led her caregivers to label her a demanding and difficult patient.

In their drive to mend a broken Humpty Dumpty, caregivers did not understand that this wounded person struggled against the negation of her essence, the negation of her personhood and identity. How else could Heather's broken self survive?

Who would listen to her speak of her confusion, despair, loss of dignity, and loss of independence? Who would understand Heather, the person who struggled to reclaim her life? Why did the caregivers refuse to stop and listen?

If the caregivers had stopped to listen, Heather's story might have guided their healing hands in helping them understand the nature of her suffering and the complexities of her care.

Heather expected her caregivers to treat her as an intelligent, thinking person. Her expectations were unmet.

Heather's grim reality was difficult to endure for she was divided into two separate halves. Her body was split down the middle. Her left side was paralyzed and her right side struggled to compensate. Her once athletic body was now deprived of balance. And she struggled to relearn how to speak.

Heather's protracted stay in the hospital imprisoned her. Yet she bravely resisted the role of dependent patient. Unable to formulate the words to express her suffering, grief pursued her. And at times, her mind was filled with thoughts of suicide.

Unmet Expectations

> *"The relief of suffering and the cure of disease must be seen as twin obligations of a medical profession that is truly dedicated to the care of the sick. Physicians' failure to understand the nature of suffering can result in medical intervention that (though technically adequate) not only fails to relieve suffering but becomes a source of suffering itself."*[18]
>
> —Dr. Eric J. Cassell

Prior to her surgery, the doctor informed Heather that her hospital stay would last five to seven postoperative days. She would then be discharged and would walk out through the hospital door.

But Heather's glioblastoma was too extensive to remove in its entirety. Despite the best of efforts of the surgical team to extricate as much as possible of the tumor from her brain, the marathon twelve-hour surgery was traumatic. Heather suffered a stroke on the operating table that paralyzed the left side of her body and destroyed her ability to speak.

All surgery carries risks. Sometimes, despite great skill, determination, and good intention, there are things that medicine simply cannot fix. And there are times when medical intervention results in greater harm and suffering for the patient.

Such was the plight of Heather. She could no longer walk and her speech was irreparably harmed. It took months before she could form words again, then countless time and effort to form even the simplest sentences. Yet within her broken body remained an artist, a musician, a once-athletic woman with a fiercely sharp wit and intellect that no one but her family could understand and appreciate.

The results of Heather's near-death stroke during surgery prolonged her stay in the acute care hospital for four and a half months and brought her endless suffering.

Heather's injured mind and body required time to heal. She had lost her sense of self. To recover from the onslaught of invasive brain surgery, surgical stroke, and the unmet expectations of physical rehabilitation, required mental and spiritual healing. Heather's convalescence necessitated an extended period of compassionate care, support, and encouragement.

In days gone by, patients convalesced in sanatoriums that sustained and nurtured them. Convalescence ensures peace and renewal of body, mind, and soul. Convalescence allows healing and recuperation.

With moral courage and loving support, and in her own good time, Heather would experience a renaissance; she would re-create herself.

Months after her traumatic surgery, and with her one functioning arm, Heather clasped her mother's hand. Her voice was slow and deliberate. Her words, no longer upside-down, reached her mother's listening ears. "I don't care about the cancer. I just want to walk. I just want to regain my independence and find meaning in my life. Father said music would help heal my soul. He said music would help me find myself. Do you think he's right?"

What did Heather need?

She needed to tell her story a hundred times or more so that others would understand Heather, the person. She needed time to heal her injured mind. The essential elements of Heather's care required courage, hope, love, and the understanding patience of able-bodied helpers.

To this Heather added, "And as well as all of that, Mother, I need laughter and more laughter. Tell me something funny, Mother. Tell me about your life."

"Mind Is the Master Power": Dora

Mind is the Master power that moulds and makes,
And Man is Mind, and evermore he takes
The tool of Thought, and, shaping what he wills,
Brings forth a thousand joys, a thousand ills: —
He thinks in secret, and it comes to pass:
Environment is but his looking-glass.[19]

—James Allen (1864–1912)

Poets and scholars write of the power of the thinking-feeling mind and its impact on the body and the soul. A person's thoughts and feelings are part of their private self. Thoughts and feelings mold and shape a happy, sad, or fearful state. The mind chatters; the body listens and responds. Notwithstanding a need to protect the private self, peace of mind comes to those who are heard and understood.

Each story in this book reveals aspects of the individual self, aspects that acknowledge the patient's experience in relation to his or her illness. Patient stories are the conveyors of knowledge that enhance patient care. Stories are products of the mind that unveil a unique and individual way of thinking. If the stories in this book were painted on canvas, they would reveal a reality of the patient's world hitherto unseen.

The mind is blessed with the capability of mental imagery, which allows us to drift into daydreams in order to plan and modify our reality. Children are masters of imagery when in rapt attention they take pleasure from a favorite story. Children enter easily into storyland where they gain knowledge, empowerment, and affirmation of themselves. The story of Stephen and his classmates illustrates how children walk with the heroes of their minds. The story of Abby and her puppet conveys the power of imagery and hope.

Vivid imaginations also serve adults. Creative visualization and meditation, for example, are known to relieve stress and distress.

Nurse Beth recalled an incident that confirmed to her the power of imagery. It occurred in a local shopping mall where two people had purchased Lotto tickets. Pocketing their tickets, a husband and wife proceeded to walk through the mall. And as they walked, they began to argue. Other shoppers overheard the argument as the couple's voices grew louder. Their energetic debate was powered by their wild imaginings of a vast lottery win. This led to a dispute as to how their winnings would be spent. Their newfound wealth was so vivid in their minds that the husband and wife were unaware of the uproar they caused.

A Hundred Thousand Ills

Dora waited at the clinic with utmost dread. She waited for treatment that overwhelmed her. In her twenty-six years of living, nothing compared with the fear she experienced on her visits to the clinic. The treatments reinforced her anguished awareness of the devastation of her illness.

Not long before, Dora herself had been a member of the clinic staff and she had coaxed patients to relax during treatments. But at that time, her work had fully occupied her mind, leaving no room to understand what it must have been like to be the patient.

Despite the onset of her illness, Dora continued her university studies. Her lessons in philosophy and the humanities gave her peace of mind during remission from her illness.

But the radiation treatments, their subsequent failure, and the progression of Dora's illness brought inner turmoil. A defeated Dora believed that her illness would result in a hospital admission. "And my family won't see me as myself. My disintegration will be complete."

Dora's mind brought forth "a thousand ills."

Dora's fears of personal "disintegration" were confirmed when her fiancé fled the scene. She was sure his desertion proved that she was "worthless."

Dora's fears gave way to hysteria, which created a full-blown crisis. Her hysteria wreaked havoc throughout the clinic, alarming patients and staff, who were scared stiff by her screams.

Dora had lost her self-control. Her suffering was intense. She was in desperate need of care and understanding.

Building a Bridge to Reach Dora

Children delight in the harmony of the human voice. Nurse Beth wondered if Dora's inner child could be reached in this time of crisis and abject fear. And she wondered if the power of imagery could release Dora from the tyranny of her mind.

Nurse Beth decided to make a move. She would talk Dora through her awful fears by acknowledging Dora's harsh reality. Beth told Dora, "You're not alone. I'm sitting here right beside you."

Nurse Beth continued to talk with Dora telling her, "Anxiety has robbed you of control. And your life seems to have lost its meaning. We need to put this right. Will you give me your trust so that together we can fix things?"

With a nod of her head, Dora accepted.

Nurse Beth used guided imagery and the power of hypnosis to help Dora achieve an altered state of deep relaxation. Autohypnosis, which was self-induced, worked to stem the turbulent flow within Dora's troubled mind. And it allowed Dora access to a reality that took on a new and different shape.

How did Dora achieve this altered state of peaceful relaxation?

Although no clinical hypnotherapist was present to facilitate the process, when Nurse Beth sat with Dora and acknowledged Dora's reality, it eased her wretched state. Nurse Beth then helped guide the process of creative visualization. But it was the power of Dora's own mind and the imagery of her new altered, peaceful thoughts that empowered this courageous young woman.

The humanity and poetry of James Allen speaks to the power of the thinking-feeling mind. His book *As a Man Thinketh*[20] offers life-sustaining hope by inviting each man and woman to discover the creative aspects of their mind and its propensity to free the troubled self.

It is not uncommon for seriously ill people to reflect upon their lives and their relationships with family and friends.

Through the process of introspection, thoughts and feelings are revealed. Introspection led Dora to close the door on her old chaotic fears and never again to venture into the gloom of self-loathing and defeat.

The impact of illness led Dora's mother and aunt to suggest that Dora devise a plan of action to replace the pursuit of cure. Both mother and aunt offered to help Dora with her plan. They understood that a positive, supportive environment alters the perception of pain.

Dora's aunt suggested, "Whenever I take my moody gloom on a walk, it soon disappears. Walking never fails to do the trick."

Dora's mother added, "You're not up to walking, Dora. But we could take you for a drive in the country. We could crack open the car widows and you'd enjoy the cool fresh air. We'll wrap you up in grandma's soft, blue shawl. You'll be nice and warm."

Grateful to her family for their devotion and care, Dora felt secure. And she enjoyed a lasting peace.

Dora made a spreadsheet that became her plan of action. She gathered up the moments in just one precious day and found that there were times when her pain was in decline. At other times, she needed quiet and restful sleep. Dora named her sleeping moments "here-and-there." But the moments that gave her untold joy were those she named "now-and-then" for those were the moments she spent in the presence of her family.

Dora went home for the remainder of her illness and during that time she lived without fear.

Like so many patients, Dora found the routine of her morning care a source of great comfort. One morning, Dora's mother and aunt held her in their arms as they rearranged the pillows. Embraced in those warm, loving arms, Dora gently died.

"Detached Compassion": Geraldine

Grief is not the enemy. Grief is not burnout.
Grief is woven into the very fabric of life.

Two events, unrelated yet entwined, dramatized the function of Dunira's hospice palliative care team and revealed its vulnerability. Geraldine's admission to Dunira coincided with the arrival of a consulting psychologist. His role was to provide support to the staff and relief from stress. His noninvolvement with patients led him to assume a clinically detached posture. Yet despite the psychologist's lack of connection with patients, he proposed that Geraldine's care be modified to be delivered with "detached compassion."

To be detached indicates disassociation, an absence of relationship. On the other hand, compassion is a feeling state that indicates humanitarian concern and personal connection.

Palliative care embraces humanity in the compassionate relief of pain and suffering. Moreover, palliative care nurtures the interdependent nature of caring relationships between patient, families, and caregivers. The concept of detachment is alien to the practice of palliation.

The presence of the consulting psychologist at Dunira Hospice was something of an anomaly, since within the team he was an observer rather than a team player. And he had no knowledge of palliative care. Acquiring knowledge of a subject takes time and personal investment. To gain understanding of the subject of one's inquiry requires more than listening and observing or referring to a textbook. The foundation of knowledge and understanding requires investing oneself in the process. In other words, understanding comes with doing.

But for the consulting psychologist, who stood apart, the hospice team became the sole subject of his investigation and inquiry.

One might argue that the psychologist was wise to stand back and observe the hospice team at work. After all it was his intention to provide them with staff support. And in order to provide staff support, he needed to know the cause of staff distress.

Unavoidably, palliative staff experience distress and grieve the loss of patients for whom they have cared. But with the arrival of the psychologist, the hospice team found itself under the close scrutiny of his ever-watchful eye. The psychologist was curious about the team's approach to patient care.

Geraldine's Intractable Pain

The aggressive nature of Geraldine's illness resulted in her admission to Dunira.

Geraldine was twenty-eight years old and her pain, out of control, was unremitting. Her plans to join the nursing service in India were forfeited when she lost her health to cancer. Pain specialists and neurological consultants tried in vain to relieve the smoldering embers of Geraldine's excruciating pain. Despite their continued efforts, her pain persisted.

Medical literature (including sources such as the *Monograph on the Management of Cancer Pain, Physician-Assisted Dying,* and *Living with Dying*) provides information on pain that cannot be relieved. These works indicate that narcotics play a significant part in the relief of advanced tumor pain. They also illustrate how narcotics in combination with other drugs and treatment modalities, including patient support, alleviate suffering. However, experts in pain management suggest that a small percentage of chronic pain cannot be adequately relieved in spite of current techniques in pain management.

Geraldine's pain belonged to that most unfortunate category.

Despite the best efforts of pain specialists and neurological consultants, Geraldine's pain raged on.

Dunira Hospice offered this courageous young woman unconditional love and support. The bond that strengthened the relationship between Geraldine and her caregivers was forged in compassion and altruistic care. When relationships are nurtured in a community of care, patients, families, and caregivers collaborate, forming a team and a bond. And within this caring environment, Geraldine bore her pain.

Geraldine had come of age in foster care. She was known by the shortened version of her name. Her friends called her Geri. And Geri she remained. Her surrogate family at Dunira welcomed her and shared her difficult journey.

With her team of caregivers, Geri was at times the younger sister, the courageous daughter, the beloved friend. Her palliative caregivers shared her pain and suffering. And in pursuit of dignified care, they sought to protect her.

A Grieving Hospice Team

Grief and suffering are woven into the fabric of meaningful relationships both in health and in sickness. In serious illness, palliative caregivers share the patient's journey. As the patient offers his or her story with the palliative team, the caregivers listen deeply, because within that story lies wisdom that can help alleviate suffering. When caregivers ask, "How are things for you right now?," they acknowledge that from moment to moment things change for the patient. The caregivers understand that within the patient's response, within their story, lies essential information to help direct their care. This ongoing, sensitive, and open-ended dialogue is a living exchange of shared humanity. And it is this communicative back and forth between patient and caregiver, this reciprocation that prevents boundaries of distance, which would otherwise erode patient care.

There are those who believe that burnout occurs when suffering is shared by caregivers. But grief is not burnout. Grief is a fundamental part of life. Grief begs to be felt, to be shared and accepted, not hidden away or suppressed. Geri's caregivers grieved because they understood the magnitude of her intractable pain yet were unable to extinguish its fire. Each of them in their own way shared the excruciating reality of Geri's pain and struggled daily with their inability to eradicate her physical suffering.

Yet without understanding the philosophy of palliative care, the consulting psychologist sought to change the nature of the relationship between Geri and her team of caregivers. He wanted them to stand back and proposed that team members adopt an "attitude of professional distance and decorum."

Subsequently, a pattern of misunderstanding, unclear com-

munication, and entanglement cascaded into unresolved issues
that simply heightened the stress of the hospice staff.

The Stone Thrower

Dunira's consulting psychologist had no knowledge of the art
of palliative care. Indeed, he might have been the thrower of
stones, who disturbed the serenity of a gentle pool. Skilled in
the knowledge of human behavior, his analytical mind focused
on the behavior of the hospice team. But he failed to understand that palliative caregivers comprise only *one* part of a
mutually dependent whole. Patients, families, and caregivers
combine their resources to form the palliative team. It is futile
to consider a palliative team without the inclusion of patients
and family as participating partners-in-care.

Relief from stress is what we crave without understanding
that the ultimate stress-free state is death. How vulnerable, how
naive, to consider that the pain of grief would simply disappear,
washed away by a psychologist skilled in stress relief. Yet for the
briefest period of time, Geri's caring team believed that relief
from stress was close at hand.

With the benefit of hindsight, such thinking made no sense
because, since the psychologist was unfamiliar with the work
and philosophy of palliative care, he remained a stranger. A
stranger on the outside, looking in.

The psychologist believed that the hospice team was over-
involved with patients and family and therefore lacked professional decorum. His belief was false since all hospice teams
are comprised of patients, family, and caregivers. To label the

palliative team as flawed and "unprofessional" because of caring relationships between patients, families, and staff negated the very essence of palliative care.

Because the psychologist was not involved with the patients or their families, how could he begin to understand the purpose and function of the team and their work? How foolish for team members to assume that he could possibly understand their grief in relation to Geri's care.

An Unusual Experience

Dunira's dayroom provided the ideal setting for the staff support group. Team members who could spare the time attended. The psychologist occupied a large reclining chair that stood with its back against the wall. The coffee table provided a discrete distance between himself and attending team members. From this strategic position in the room, the psychologist faced his subjects.

The psychologist employed many tactics and strange practices during his sessions on stress relief. Using games that he had designed to mold and shape the mind, he hoped to change the staff's "unprofessional" behavior.

But how could his games possibly "cure" Geri's caregivers of their grief in relation to Geri's care and her intractable pain? And what did he have in mind when he placed an *invisible hippopotamus* in front of them on the coffee table?

The psychologist's rules for relieving stress seemed outlandish and extreme.

"Rule number one," the psychologist told them, "before you

say one word, pick up that *invisible hippopotamus* and hold it in your lap."

Rule number one led to a protracted silence. Tension filled the room until someone finally pretended to pick up that invisible hippo, then stumbled verbally through some foolish words. But what could a frazzled caregiver possibly say as she struggled to break the deadly silence that hung over the room?

In the presence of a hippopotamus that was invisible and a psychologist who was silent, an intelligent discussion seemed impossible. Was silence a means of controlling staff?

In the flash of an instant and despite the familiar surroundings of their workplace, the group of mature palliative caregivers suddenly felt incompetent and inadequate. The invisible hippopotamus had served no other purpose than to increase the distress of the hospice staff.

If behavior modification was the essence of stress relief, team members decided to abstain. Perhaps an invisible hippo can provide the means to identify problems that impair the functioning of the mind. And if a psychologist employs the process of free association of thoughts, images, and experimentation to achieve a change in behavior, that is well and good. But palliative care is *not* about behavior that requires modification in order to establish control over staff. Why then offer such a procedure to hospice staff in the name of "support"?

And so it was that the stone-throwing consulting psychologist thought to change the method and delivery of humanistic care at Dunira. "Detached compassion" was his psychological aim. He didn't understand when hospice staff expressed their feelings of inadequacy, anger, fear, and despair at their inability to ease Geri's immense physical suffering. Instead, he viewed those feeling states as character flaws and sought to change them through his version of behavior modification.

But the members of Dunira's hospice team remained incorrigible. And their behavior resisted the psychologist's intended modification. The hospice caregivers understood what the psychologist failed to grasp: grief is normal; grief is not a character flaw. It is humanly impossible to care deeply for someone who is suffering and not grieve for that person and his or her pain. The hospice caregivers understood that grief was part of their job. And they understood that the only way to handle the "stress" of their grief over Geri was to share that grief openly, to talk about it, to laugh and cry, and to support one another with camaraderie and community. The palliative team would take care of Geri, and they would take care of one another too.

"Have we lost our sense of humor?"

Judy, the occupational therapist from "Down Under," set the record straight for her caregiver colleagues. The audacity of her words reverberated round the lunchroom. And like a refreshing spray of cool water, splashed the face of every person seated around the lunchroom table.

Judy's Australian accent rang out. "Have we lost our sense of humor? That daft sod thought he could change the way we care for our patients! That *detached compassion* of his was designed to change the "*shape*" of things all right. Who does he think he is? Director of some psychodrama? Come on. Take a look at this table. We've got yummy treats, chocolates, homemade Christmas shortbread. Let's pig out! 'Cause eating's the only thing that's going to change *our shape*! And I'm not sharing any of this with that dumb clone of Dr. Freud."

Brenda, who gave hours of her time as a volunteer, chimed in, "Maybe the psychologist was trying to save us from burnout."

"Ha!" Judy exclaimed. "Think again, girl. It was more than burnout that caused our stress. Think of the weight of that bloody big hippopotamus sitting in your lap!"

Sister Beatrice laughed. "Would it have made any difference if Mr. Psychologist had used an Australian kangaroo instead?"

"Not bloody likely," Judy quipped. "Hippopotamus. Dragon. Kangaroo. Makes not one bit of difference 'cause that psychologist hung a label 'round our necks. We're just a bunch of "*unprofessionals*" as far as he's concerned."

Laughter brought relief to the team of weary caregivers.

In her Irish brogue Sister Beatrice announced, "Well, I for one will not be wasting my time with any more of that so-called stress relief. Better by far for you and me to sit quietly with our Geri."

How did a psychologist and a caring hospice team come to lock horns, creating barriers that got in the way?

First and foremost, a lack of understanding of the nature of palliative care placed the psychologist in a no-win situation. Secondly, his model of "detached compassion" would have prevented the humanistic relationship between team members. Sadly, with no investment of himself, nor any understanding of the interpersonal relationships of trust between patients, family, and caregivers, the psychologist remained an outsider.

Two schools of thought had clashed. On the one hand, compassion and benevolence in the art of palliation. And on the other hand, clinical and professional separation. That clash destroyed the tranquility of the palliative care unit. Those two opposing concepts were in contradiction and for a time they disturbed the functioning of the hospice team.

The administration of the acute care hospital had intervened by hiring the consulting psychologist to provide Dunira with staff support. But lacking an understanding of the nature of palliative care, how palliative caregivers walk *toward* the seriously ill, not away from them, the intervention, as well-intentioned as it was, smacked of amateur meddling.

The psychologist did not understand the role of the palliative caregiver as one of bridging the emotional gulf that separates the living from the dying. It would be near impossible to connect at that junction if one of the team was "detached," obscured by some distant, professional role.

Grief, moreover, is not a sickness of the mind. Grief and loss are realities that each of us must face on our journey through life. And as members of Dunira's hospice team, we were vulnerable, as strong only as the weakest link in our caring, communicating chain.

A Time of Good Cheer

As a member of Dunira's hospice team, I shared the reality of Geri's suffering.

It was Christmas Eve, and in a daze I walked to the cathedral for the evening service. Along the way, I saw a blind beggar. She stood on the corner of Smithers and Main. I was warmed by the presence of this serene woman, who, despite the bitter wind, uttered not a single word of complaint. Music from her simple barrel organ filled the street with sounds of Christmas past. But Geri was in my thoughts every step of the way.

The cathedral teemed with people full of bright Christmas cheer. The brass band of the Salvation Army played music lofty and high. But to me the scene was unreal. All I could think of was Geri; her presence consumed my thoughts as if the two of us were alone, huddled together apart from the scene. A soprano, young and elegant, lifted her voice and sang the hymn, "Abide with Me." But I heard not a word of that hymn for I had fallen into a deep, dark pool of grief. I wept for the blind woman. And I wept for the folks who stood in a queue without cheer, waiting for a handout of food.

I wept for Geri. And I wept for me.

Just an hour had passed since leaving Geri's hospice room. What words had that psychologist used? "Detached compassion." Such empty, meaningless words. Yet his words consumed me.

Just one hour earlier, the psychologist had stood outside Geri's room and witnessed a scene that to his eyes was absurd and "unprofessional."

What the psychologist had witnessed as I sat on Geri's bed was Geri's hand pressed close to my chest. But what the psychologist did not understand was that Geri's hand on my chest registered the rhythm of my breathing. He did not understand that the rhythm and sound of my breath helped Geri slow things down. He did not understand that as Geri and I breathed together, Geri's own rapid, shallow gasps for air steadied and eased her fear.

The psychologist failed to understand that breathing together with Geri was but a simple palliative act of compassion, comfort, and care for a young woman in extreme pain and fear.

When I left Geri's room, the psychologist blocked my way to admonish me.

"To be effective," he scolded, "you must maintain a stance that is discrete. You must retain a professional distance from your patients."

And in anger, I swallowed my rage.

The psychologist knew nothing of Geri. He had not even entered Geri's room, much less witnessed her raw despair. Nor was he aware of the suffocating odor of sickness that filled her room and clung to Geri's body like a tattered shroud. Closed drapes held out all light. Nothing but the sound of Geri's rasping breath broke the silence of her room.

Nor did the psychologist hear Geri's cry: "I have so much pain! Don't they believe me?"

"Yes," I told Geri. "Yes, they believe you. At this very moment Dr. Daniel, Claire, the pharmacist, and the neurologist, they're all working towards a plan to ease your pain. And I'm here to stay with you now, Geri."

"But where are they? I need to know their plan! Tell them to hurry. I feel like Job."

In anguish, Geri pleaded with me, "Please. Stay, breathe with me."

But it was impossible to keep up with Geri's rapid, chaotic breath.

"Geri, darling," I said. "I'm all out of puff trying to keep up with you. Tell you what. I'll sit here on your bed. Press your hand against my chest. Now feel the rhythm of my breathing. That's it. We'll breathe together. Hold on, Geri. That's my girl. Your breathing's getting easier, Geri."

When next she spoke, Geri asked me, "Can you feel the

power of God in this room? God is here! God is here with me now and he is wrapping up my pain."

A few moments later, Judy, the occupational therapist, tiptoed into the room. She carried a book and a vase of old-fashioned Sweet William. Geri's fondness of those flowers lay in their rainbow of colors, in the strength of their tiny floral heads clustered in groups as if for protection. Judy set the flowers down on the bedside table where Geri would see them when she woke.

Then in a whisper, Judy said, "Geri looks so peaceful when she sleeps. I'll stay here now. And Beatrice plans to stay the night."

In the early hours of Christmas morning, Nurse Marty reached me by phone.

Marty's words were simple. "God wrapped up Geri's pain. Beatrice and I sat with her during those quiet hours before dawn. Geri remained peaceful and lucid. We prayed together, and she whispered good-bye. Her death was gentle."

Like nature's change of seasons, death is a release that causes us to pause. And with the birth of spring, nature brings us hope for the continuation of life.

The Coming of Spring

Spring arrived with a cacophony of sound that filled the valley with the roar of white thunder. The river gave up its solid state as boulders of ice ripped apart and floated swiftly downstream. Anxious residents, with sandbags at the ready, waited for the fury to subside. Not for the first time, the river burst its banks, flooding nearby houses on its low-lying shore. In the city, melting ice ran in rivulets as winter released its icy grip. And with boundless joy, children squished through muddy puddles of slushy snow. In no time at all, scarves and mittens would be relegated to winter's deep, forgotten closet.

Violet's Anguish

Violet believed that the birth of springtime would bring her joy. It would be just like the old days when she and Roger had laughed their way through the trials of married life. Soon they would celebrate the completion of Roger's achievements, his PhD, a doctorate of philosophy. All the difficulties they had faced during the long winter months would be of no lasting consequence.

Roger had been full of doubt when Violet toiled with extra work to pay his university fees. She willingly undertook the onerous task of a heavy workload because she believed that no sacrifice was too great for Roger. But winter and work had taken its toll. And Violet lost her health. She became so thin that winter's chill seeped into her fragile bones. The oncologist confirmed leukemia.

Unable to cope, Roger withdrew. Violet, alone and consumed by loneliness, sought comfort from her priest.

Roger's studies absorbed him. He never spoke of his wife's illness, nor did he share his feelings with anyone. And Violet faced the trauma of her life-threatening illness alone.

Florence Nightingale revealed the reality and solitary nature of illness, so often misunderstood, with her words:

> "How little the real sufferings of illness are known and understood. How little does any one in good health fancy him or even herself into the life of a sick person."[21]

These poignant words of wisdom are an appeal for compassion, autonomy, and dignity to alleviate the suffering of the sick.

Violet longed to talk with Roger about their uncertain future. She yearned to be held in a gentle, loving embrace.

But when had it happened, this absence of touch? How could the caring comfort of touch, once so reassuring, so confirming, have simply disappeared?

Violet wondered if she was to blame. Illness, medical appointments, and treatment procedures had robbed her of time to spend with Roger. But Roger was fully occupied with academic work, so much so that he hardly noticed her absence. The anguish of her solitude was more than Violet could bear. Why was Roger unwilling to share her fearful journey?

When fear of blood transfusions left Violet weak and sick, the caring staff at the clinic reached out to her and said, "Now don't you fret, Violet. This blood was donated by a big, strong lumberjack from Quebec. And this gift of life-giving energy was meant just for you."

But Roger's once familiar voice remained silent. His communication in one-syllable words disarmed Violet.

Desperate to reach her husband, Violet pleaded. "Roger, why won't you look at me?" But Roger stayed silent.

"Roger, we don't spend any time together."

Finally, Roger replied. "Medical appointments take up all of your time. And I'm busy with studies that I'm doing for you. There's a professorship for me when I'm finished. That means you won't have to return to work. You can stay at home. Take it easy."

So that was it?

Did Roger really believe his words?

Violet's energy quickly vanished. She talked, but Roger could not hear. It was as if Roger inhabited another world. Talking takes energy, especially when talking gets you nowhere. Silent tension grew between them.

Violet saw in Roger's eyes a reflection of herself as a person from his past. Roger's voice was distant. It reached her from afar. Roger spoke with an unnerving calm that pierced her heavy heart.

With callous cruelty, Roger brushed Violet aside when he said, "I don't know what you want from me. Your demands are unrealistic. As for loving you, I'm still here. Isn't that enough?"

What anguish is wrought when love is denied, when tenderness is cast aside.

Violet asked, "How can love die?"

And then with the briefest of sighs, she added, "Oh how Roger hates it when I sigh."

Violet's suffering was endless. The old ways were gone, and she could not reclaim them. But when faced with serious illness, what person would choose to separate from an unloving spouse? Violet was thirty-nine years old and she was fatally ill. In the process of reviewing her life, she acknowledged that her marriage to Roger was a union in name only. Violet shared the anguish of her soul with Beth, her palliative nurse and friend.

Beth heard Violet say, "I'm Catholic. I don't believe in divorce. I understand there's good and bad in married life. Sometimes we bring out the worst in each other. I always thought that when we listened and shared our hurts, we chased the blues away. But when Roger turns away in silence, I know the bad is here to stay. Silence is the awful reality that exists between us. That silence makes me ill. And I feel helpless."

Violet reached into the drawer of the bedside table and pulled out a photograph of Roger. She handed the photo to Beth and said, "Stick this picture on the wall because I'm going to throw darts at it."

Nurse Beth took the photograph. "Violet, you are worth so much more. Roger doesn't deserve you." Then she asked, "Do you think Roger is playing the part of Peter Pan? The boy who refused to grow up?"

Peter Pan, a children's hero, dwells in the land of make-believe. Yet perhaps Peter Pan represents the universal fear of growing up, of taking responsibility, of being adult, of dealing with the fear of life and death, of not hiding from the grim reality of a spouse's terminal illness. Nurse Beth had given Violet a hook on which to hang her pain.

Thinking out loud, Violet said, "Roger's behavior is unbelievable. He's just not in touch with reality."

"So should we send Roger to London, England, to Kensington Gardens?" Beth responded in humor. "Roger could visit the statue of Peter Pan, make a 'study' of it. Maybe it'd enlighten him. You never know, he might just recognize himself."

But where had Roger gone? Someone bearing his likeness had taken his place, and that someone was a stranger. From his lofty ivory tower, Roger looked down on the rest of the world. Appalled by Violet's illness, he had turned his back and walked away. His detachment lacked compassion and revealed that he had already set foot on a new and different path. He took all his scholarly learning and headed off, far away from his dying wife.

The impact of an uncaring marriage on the seriously ill is profound. A broken union, a breakdown in communication, a spouse or partner who walks away, exacerbates suffering. As caring and supportive as the palliative team is, it has no magic to mend the broken heart of a dying patient. But what they, and caring friends, can offer is compassionate presence, a listening, nonjudgmental ear, and an empathetic heart to relieve some of the patient's grief and anguish.

Violet was unable to cope with Roger's departure. For her, the dissolution of their marriage was profound. Violet knew no peace as feelings of anger and betrayal besieged her mind.

Violet could not accept that Roger had left her far behind. Overwhelmed with a sense of defeat, she swallowed her anger, and it festered in despair.

Why did Roger fail to see that his once beloved wife had lost hope?

Roger and Violet were both out of touch, out of reach.

Locked inside his academia, Roger left behind a foundation that was broken and in decay. Yet not so long before that very same foundation had supported and sustained his life.

Abandoned by her husband in her time of greatest need, a sense of betrayal consumed Violet's mind and robbed her of any peace. Throughout her troubled dreams and waking moments, children's faces haunted her. Their childish voices floated in the air, and Violet could hear the anguish of their innocence lost. And all the while, betrayal filled her mind and robbed her peace.

Full of despair, Violet grew weary of her broken life. As her two longstanding friends kept vigil at her side, Violet summoned her dignity and said a final good-bye.

Roger may never know that Violet's stature was immense and would forever remain in the minds of her many friends. For Violet left a legacy of compassion and enduring love. Abused children of all ages would long remember her, for it was Violet who had worked to set them free.

Harry and Mabel's Acceptance

Down at the clinic, the doctor had told Harry that he would not survive the winter. Now it was spring and as long as he could stay at home, Harry was not afraid of dying.

Harry told Nurse Beth, "My nurses have taken care of my pain. But it's the nausea and this awful tiredness that gets me down. Mind you, I've been lucky, 'cause now at the end of the road Mabel's by my side. She's taking good care of me. My Mabel is the salt of the earth. But when I'm gone, she'll need to put her God-given talents to better use."

Harry was not a man to mince words. In fact, some considered him cantankerous for he could be sharp, outspoken, and blunt when required. But Harry was at his best when he described his adventures at sea. Harry was a fisherman who delighted in telling stories about his wife, Mabel. She was Harry's first-class mate, always there to lend a hand.

Harry told of the "many times I was forced to tie Mabel to the boat, lest a sudden squall should sweep her overboard. She was just a slip of a girl, my Mabel. And full of adventure. Mabel loved the sea and could gut a salmon as fast as any fisherman."

The sea had been Harry's life until cancer took hold of him. Strange how cancer could take hold of a person, without anybody knowing from where it had come. But Harry didn't spend time wondering where his cancer had come from. Mostly, he wondered where he would have been if the cancer had not taken hold. Harry believed that "The little guy can no longer make a living from the sea 'cause the big fishing companies have done 'em in." According to Harry, "Those big fishing fleets sweep the sea with greed, scooping up huge quantities of salmon. And those noble salmon don't stand a chance. Herring stocks are down. And those new-fangled fish farms are a disaster."

Harry told Nurse Beth, "My cancer has saved me from becoming obsolete. 'Cause where would I be now? Most likely, I'd be relegated to the scrap heap. A dinosaur. A relic of the past. Maybe I'd be on welfare and social assistance. For sure I'd be a fisherman without any work."

Harry loved to give Mabel advice. If only she would take it to heart and put her talents to better use. Harry believed that the owner of the local craft shop exploited Mabel.

But Mabel, clinging to her independence, said, "It's not

what Harry thinks or feels about my knitting buffalo-wool jackets. What matters is how I feel. It's good for my health and keeps me sane. I sell the jackets on consignment. The owner of the shop takes his percentage. I make enough money to buy more wool. Don't get paid for my work. But I feel good creating something useful. And my jackets sell real quick 'cause they're popular. I'm kinda isolated taking care of Harry. But when I work with that wonderful, soft wool, it's like a vacation."

Mabel paused for a moment, then added, "It was only in those nighttime dreams that I got lost. But, Anna, my friend, put me right on that score."

Mabel described her wise friend Anna, whose father was the chief of a First Nations band. Anna helped Mabel understand the meaning of those scary nighttime dreams.

"Mabel, can't you see? Your dreaming mind is busy with the worry work of grief."

Anna was right. Mabel was worrying, grieving silently about her husband's cancer. Anna gave Mabel a little pillow filled with fragrant herbs. "Let the hops and herbs in this pillow lead your mind to nature's garden. It'll fill your senses. And your mind will find peace."

Anna also taught Mabel to mend the broken strands of the soft, thick buffalo wool that Mabel used to knit her jackets. Then Mabel showed Nurse Beth what she had learned from Anna, how to join the broken strands and make the join invisible. Mabel placed two strands side by side and, with the thumbs and index fingers of both hands, rubbed gently until the separate strands formed a perfect, invisible join. Almost like magic and yet so simple.

Mabel told Nurse Beth, "Anna is my true friend. My spirit guide. But she's going back home to her reserve in the North."

Anna was leaving, and soon Mabel would be faced with another loss.

Mabel had packed a lot of living into her full, yet short life. She coped with her fears and her grief in small attentive ways—through her nature dreams and spirit dreams, sharing openly with her dear friend, Anna, and from broken strands making invisible mends.

Despite the harsh conditions of her life, Mabel never once regarded herself as a victim. For as her husband, Harry, liked to say, "Life's a challenge. The bad experiences help us remember the times that were good."

Secure in the comfort of his home, his family at his side, and with the support of palliative care, Harry was not crippled by the fear of isolation or the fear of uncontrolled pain. Harry had Mabel. And they were soul mates. They supported each other. Fisherman and fisherwoman, they had shared life's adventure. At times, hardship had dogged their path. Yet with determination and courage, they had endured.

When Harry was diagnosed with cancer, he confronted it head-on. Illness was one of life's events, one of those challenges that helped Harry remember the good times.

Harry's storytelling gift of adventures at sea, coupled with the belief that cancer had saved him from welfare and unemployment, were Harry's ways of dealing with illness. And by so doing, Harry refused an identity he loathed, the identity of becoming obsolete.

Through to the conclusion of his life, Harry remained true to himself, a fisherman, first and foremost.

A Catalog of Labels

abels identify and provide information. Labels can also guide and direct responses that in turn motivate behavior. Meg Brodie paid little attention to labels, especially those that identified her as brazen and self-assured—a *gallus besom* in Scottish slang. Endowed with wisdom and common sense, Meg was, without doubt, streetwise and self-reliant. A daughter of the thistle, Meg's personality was audacious, as warm and colorful as the heather in the land of her birth.

Meg's Story

Amongst her many admirable qualities, Meg was a diva of fashion. But the outfits she sported were a reflection of her personality and seldom if ever copied by others.

Meg stood five feet two inches tall and sixty-two years young. Meg's husband, Malcolm, the Boss, or the Gaffer as Meg called him, did not approve of her high sense of fashion. Dressed in an oyster-colored, long, knit top, a black lace skirt hiked well above her chubby knees, legs adorned in gray wool leggings, and on her feet a pair of black, silver-buckled brogues, Meg presented herself to the world. With a face bright and shiny, old, and full of mirth, she was more leprechaun than fashion model. But everyone at Dunira Hospice loved Meg for it was as if her mere presence ushered in the warm smiling sun.

Malcolm Brodie, the Gaffer, was admitted to Dunira Hospice following an extensive period of sickness. His care at home had been provided by the palliative home care team and his dedicated wife, Meg. Meg's commitment to caring for Malcolm at home was never in any doubt, but her doctor had intervened and persuaded her to consider respite hospice care. Malcolm's stay at Dunira Hospice was of short duration.

One day and armed with two cups of steaming black coffee, Meg marched into the social worker's office and set the two cups down.

Jean looked up and said, "Meg Brodie, it is yourself."

"Aye it's me, come t' ask a favor."

"Sit yourself down, Meg, and let me hear your pleasure."

Meg slumped down with a long sigh. "It's Malcolm," she said, "he's just thrown in the towel and died. And I'm in need of your help, Jean. *Instant disposal.* That's what I've got in mind. Oh, listen to me I can't seem t' stop talking."

Anxiety and agitation wove through Meg's rushed words. "I'm away to Vegas in a week. With enough cash to pay for Maggie and me. And to think the Gaffer doesn't know a thing about it! It's hard to believe the Gaffer's gone."

The social worker sipped her coffee and listened quietly, for it was obvious that Meg sorely needed to share her story.

"You know, my neighbors thought our Malcolm was a saint," Meg's words rushed on. "He always knew when to turn on the charm. Even charmed strangers. Always the gallant gentleman. I think the neighbors felt sorry for him. They thought I was weird. But our neighbors didn't know a thing. To them I was just a *gallus besom*. Yes, Malcolm turned on the charm for the ladies. Mind you, in his own house it was something else. There were times I thought he was the Earl of Yon Dark Place. The Devil himself. But I never did badmouth him."

Meg paused to catch her breath. "So if it's all the same t' you, Jean, I'll have instant disposal. Something simple. Will you give me a wee hand, Jean?"

The social worker extended her hand to Meg.

"Yes, Meg. I'll do what I can. Everything'll be fine. Enjoy your life and your trip to Vegas. And Meg, stay just the way you are, flawed and loveable, unique and perfect in nearly every way."

Meg smiled at Jean with obvious relief and gratitude, then added, "Are we no the daft ones? For it's no coffee we should be drinking. We should be having a wee dram to celebrate my new life."

Conditioned by forty years of marriage to Malcolm Brodie, it could be said that Meg was a downtrodden wife. The marvel of Meg's survival was her joy and love of life. Hidden from Malcolm Brodie was Meg's secret self. Her unique style of dress signified her inner rebellion, while hiding her vulnerability. Yet it had earned her the label of "*gallus besom*" and the disdain of her neighbors.

But Meg was not a brazen, self-assured, and self-absorbed woman; she was a woman of compassion, honesty, and mirth. Following the death of her husband, she sought the services of Dunira's social worker, Jean. Meg's request for "instant disposal" was simply her way of asking Jean to walk her through the steps of cremation for her deceased husband.

Meg told Jean she planned to visit Vegas with Maggie, her lifelong friend. Some might be shocked at Meg's behavior. Just one week after her husband's death, she would be on her way to Vegas. But Meg honored her newfound freedom more than any imposed cultural values.

Meg revealed a glimpse of her secret self as she took her leave of Jean. "From here on in," Meg said, "I shall be deaf to the voice of admonition and scorn. And blind will I be to those disdainful icy looks. And as well as all that, I will dance a fine jig between Heaven and Hell!"

Meg needed to let Dunira's social worker know that she was ready to face the future. With her silver-buckled shoes firmly on the ground, Meg would go her merry way. And all along that way she would sprinkle her infectious joy.

Roberta's Story

There are times when labels identify and serve to promote vulnerability in an underprivileged minority. Such was the situation for Roberta.

At the age of fourteen, Roberta acquired the label of schizophrenic. Labeled mentally ill, she was known only by her symptoms rather than her name. There were those who responded to Roberta as if she were merely an object to be pitied.

Harry, the fisherman, understood the negative effect of labeling people. He believed that illness protected him from acquiring the label of "obsolete."

To be labeled mentally ill at the age of fourteen reinforced Roberta's solitude. She was *one-of-them* rather than *one-of-us*. And in response, Roberta withdrew. Roberta occupied a private, secret world of her own creation. And within that private world she coped. The reality of Roberta's unseen world was something many did not understand.

"ROBERTA, ARE YOU HIDING?"

Roberta was admitted to Dunira Hospice from a sheltered home for the mentally ill. The information that followed her to palliative care was sparse. Her medical history revealed the onset of mental illness in early adolescence. Schizophrenia was the label assigned. It was a label that dishonored Roberta and robbed her of her personhood. Her medical record detailed her symptoms and treatment objectives. But treating the symptoms of illness is only *one* part of caring for a person who is unwell.

In the medical information provided to her palliative caregivers, Roberta's identity was nowhere to be found, there was nothing of her individuality, nothing of Roberta the person. What was documented was that at the age of twenty-four Roberta had developed cancer.

Dunira's hospice team had taken it in turn to sit by Roberta's bed and share her silence. On occasions, silence filled the room with a dreaded hush, as if waiting for some unseen danger to pass. At other times, Roberta's silence revealed her absent presence.

Was she in hiding? If Roberta was in hiding, she asked for nothing. It may well have been that she gained comfort from the peaceful presence of other patients and hospice volunteers.

By way of offering her support and reassurance, the head nurse sat by Roberta's bed and gently asked, "Roberta, what would you like from us? What can we do for you? Can we make things better than they are?"

Roberta did not respond.

Claire continued, "I'd like to tell you about Dunira. And then you might find some questions of your own. Dunira is a place where people care about one another. It's rather like a family, where we help to ease the burden of being ill. Dunira's a safe place. Sometimes we share stories, listen to music, or just spend quiet time together. But most of all, we try to chase pain out the door. If you would chose to speak, Roberta, would you talk to me and tell me where you are? And if you felt scared would you tell me? Cause if you're scared, I'd like to help chase away your fear."

Claire stopped and checked that Roberta's oxygen was in place.

"I'd love to hear from you, Roberta. It would help us know how you're feeling. Things get easier when we work together. When we're sick, it's good to have others around who care."

Silent herself now, Claire remained sitting by Roberta's bed. And she thought of what Roberta's response might be to what she'd said. But how could Claire know what Roberta's response might be? No matter what Claire thought, it would simply be a supposition since Roberta was unresponsive to everything that Claire had said.

Claire understood that searching for clues sometimes revealed something hidden. She also understood that she did not have the right to strip away the veil that shielded Roberta from intrusion. That was not Claire's intention.

Palliative care did not have a road map to guide the care of a patient suffering from an illness called schizophrenia. At Dunira, Roberta's label of schizophrenia did not count; it was meaningless to her palliative caregivers. Indeed, their greater need was to understand Roberta the person.

Head Nurse Claire disliked labels, because they created distance between people. Claire remembered the label that had identified each member of the hospice team as "unprofessional." That label had been awarded to them by a clinical psychologist who had no understanding of the nature of suffering, nor any comprehension of the grief that comes from broken bonds.

Claire continued to sit quietly with Roberta, hoping that in time, Roberta would feel secure enough to give her trust to the caregivers at Dunira.

TRUST BESTOWED

Throughout the eleven short days of Roberta's stay in palliative care, she remained silent and peaceful. The eleventh day marked a change.

The corridor at Dunira was empty and soundless. Roberta stood in the corridor alone, pressed against the wall, no slippers on her feet, no robe to keep her warm. Not a single word passed Roberta's lips, but the ice-cold grip of her fingers on Jean's arm let Jean know that Roberta was there. The stillness in Roberta's face was profound, yet her eyes compelled Jean forward, willing her to be a crutch. Jean opened her arms to Roberta and gently led the way. They staggered past Roberta's room, where her nasal prongs of oxygen lay strewn across the bed. The corridor seemed endless, no other soul in sight.

They reached the garden on the roof of the hospice and saw the fig tree waiting. With arms outstretched it beckoned, waiting to engulf Roberta, to welcome her, to hide her. A gentle rain was falling and its sweet, soft fragrance filled their senses. Still supported by Jean, Roberta turned her head and looked directly at the social worker, her eyes inviting Jean to enter her private world.

Roberta had lost her fear.

Jean hugged Roberta close and broke her fall as together they slipped to the floor. And there on the floor, raindrops splashing their skin, Roberta, still cradled in Jean's arms, slipped away and died.

Wanting only to respect the silence of Roberta, the peacefulness of the moment, Jean tapped the floor with the heel of her shoe to call for help. Head Nurse Claire and Dr. Daniel came quickly. And with the utmost of care, they laid Roberta down.

What was remarkable about Roberta's waiting by the office door for Jean, was that Roberta was expressing a strong personal choice. Roberta knew that Jean arrived late on Wednesdays for the family support group. Roberta's wait by Jean's door signaled her silent declaration that she had joined the team, a declaration confirmed by allowing the social worker to support her and then inviting Jean to enter her private world.

Roberta's declaration gave the palliative care team a sense of peace; we had not failed this courageous young woman. We had reached out to Roberta, while respecting her individuality and personhood. And Roberta had reached back.

Memorial services held at Dunira honored those who had died and offered comfort to bereaved families and caregivers.

Sister Beatrice conducted the memorial service for Roberta. The eulogy was a gracious poem that captured Roberta's ethereal self:

"*Do not stand at my grave and weep,*
I am not there; I do not sleep.
I am a thousand winds that blow.
I am the diamond glints on snow.
I am the sun on ripened grain.
I am the gentle autumn rain.
When you awaken in the morning's hush
I am the swift uplifting rush
Of quiet birds in circling flight.
I am the soft stars that shine at night.
Do not stand at my grave and cry,
I am not there; I did not die."[22]

—Mary E. Frye (1905–2004)

"Miracles" of Technology

In pursuit of cure,
medical science has neglected
to wed the healing duality of cure and care.

I never knew her name. But through a gap in the hospital screen I saw her anguish. She was old and frail. A mask of oxygen partly covered her parchment face and strands of damp white hair fell across her eyes. She had undergone a "miracle" and survived. Her family and her doctor looked like sentries. As if on guard, they stood around her bed. In soothing tones they talked to her as if she were a sickly child.

Could they not hear her anguish?

"Why did you bring me back again? Why didn't you let me die? Don't you know it's my time to go?"

They ignored her plaintiff cry and told her, "Hush!"

Medical intervention had triumphed over the calamity of an old woman's silent, lifeless heart. Skillfully, her doctors had forced that broken heart to resume its beating. They had given her drugs to stop the crushing pain. But left behind was the unknown anguish of an old woman whose story had been silenced.

Yet it is a person's story, their *Book of Life*, which reveals the places where sufferings' unattended presence lurks and hides.

Deep listening to the story of a person's life conveys realities that challenge, capture, and invite inquiring minds into the reality and the meaning of another's suffering.

Throughout my life, I have entertained the thought that hospitals resemble sterile factories, where bodies are treated with tubes and needles, drugs and technology. A place where "miracles" are manufactured and second chances are offered as packaged deals.

Yet in its aggressive pursuit of cure, medical science has neglected to wed the healing duality of cure and care. Surely the exclusion of care, in the sole pursuit of cure, serves only to negate and prolong human suffering.

The old woman behind the hospital screen was a victim of unwanted medical intervention. She was the victim of cure over care.

Triumph over adversity is achieved through awareness, compassion, and meaningful action. An old woman had begged to have her voice heard, to tell her story, but she was hushed. Fellow travelers in pursuit of humanistic care take heed for important information was ignored, negated, and silenced.

During the final days of his life, Anatole Broyard, literary critic and author, presented humanity with a gift of wisdom, when in compassion he wrote:

> "A hospital is full of wonderful and terrible stories, and if I were a doctor I would read them as one reads good fiction and let them educate me."[23]

Social Dilemmas

At the end of her life, an old woman had cried, "Why didn't you let me die? Don't you know it's my time to go?" Prolonged suffering had led the old woman to welcome death, but medical technology had delayed her dying.

Individuals with chronic pain, irreversible or terminal illness seek alleviation of their suffering from humanity's healers, our doctors. Medicine is capable of extending life. But surely in extending life, medical practitioners are morally responsible to soothe suffering at life's furthest shores.

The philosopher Peter Koestenbaum points the way when he says that:

> "We are a society at middle age, incapable of handling the philosophical problem of meaninglessness. We seek additional technology when what we need is deeper understanding of ourselves."[24]

In health and in sickness, meaninglessness is the embodiment of human suffering.

Without awareness of the impact of suffering that is endured by the seriously ill, the role of the caregiver is reduced to that of an outsider, a dispassionate observer.

But if we step *towards* the seriously ill, if we open our hearts with compassion, we can ask, "Tell me what would improve things for you right now? What was it like before things got so bad? How can you and I and all of us make things better than they are?"

And in listening with open hearts to the patients' response of what it is like for them at every moment, we can begin to understand the reality of their isolation and their pain—the nature of their suffering. This is what it means to "walk the patient's way."

Koestenbaum illuminates the philosophical aspect of humanity's deep need for connection when he writes:

> "Commitment means that I feel connected with the world. My life is experienced whole rather than fragmented."[25]

In seeking answers to a dying person's desire to hasten death, are we as a society without blame?

And if we are to blame for our lack of understanding of the suffering of others, could it be that the real culprit is our own fearful and neurotic anxiety about death?

As society grapples with the value of human life in the face of meaningless suffering, let us be aware lest a moral judgment condemns those who wish to end their life.

Euthanasia and Physician-Assisted Dying

Euthanasia and physician-assisted dying raise important moral and ethical principles regarding the philosophy of medicine. Discussions that support or oppose this "death by plan" involve the nature of human existence, the quality of patient care, and principles of morality.

While an in-depth discussion of euthanasia and physician-assisted dying is beyond the scope of this book, the controversy surrounding the ideology of assisted death nonetheless affects palliative caring.[8]

8. See also the chapter, *Dunira Hospice: Rite of Passage.*

The latent manifestations of euthanasia and physician-assisted dying have served to enhance public awareness of the humanitarian principles of palliative care. At first sight, this appears to be contradictory. Yet it is clear that decisions and laws enacted in the Netherlands and in the state of Oregon have led to the enhanced availability of palliative care services within those jurisdictions.

In the state of Oregon, application to terminate one's life requires the consensus of two physicians, confirmation of a terminal illness, and a life expectancy of no more than six months. When the above conditions have been met and the application is approved, lethal drugs are prescribed by the patient's attending physician. The patient must be of sound mind and be able to self-administer the prescribed drugs. In the state of Oregon, "Physician-assisted suicide accounts for far less than 1 percent of deaths."[26]

Surely euthanasia and physician-assisted dying is a social paradox, since the ethical and moral values of society endorse the belief that it is unlawful to terminate life. Yet society willingly condemns young men, women, and children to death during times of war.

Paradoxically, when life is without meaning or dignity, because pain and suffering is never-ending, most jurisdictions regard the termination of life as an illegal criminal act.

Thomasma and Graber, authors of the book *Euthanasia: Toward an Ethical Social Policy*, portray the manifestation of unattended, unexamined suffering in terminal illness.[27] With clarity of vision, they denounce the immorality and unethical aspects of the negation of suffering and advocate a humanitarian approach to end-of-life care.

The ideology of euthanasia is the relief of pain and suffering through a merciful death. Yet physician-assisted dying creates a moral and ethical dilemma, because the questions embedded in the teachings of spiritual values remain unanswered. In contrast, palliative care seeks the restoration of the human spirit through compassionate care and the alleviation of suffering. These two ideologies are separate and distinct. However, there are those who believe that both ideologies embrace the principle of mercy.

In 1992, Derek Humphry published a suicide manual, entitled *Final Exit*. The manual represents a lonely, desolate journey at life's conclusion. Humphry's manual has no bearing on, nor any similarity to palliative care. Yet paradoxically, what is written in *Final Exit* promotes awareness of the *need* for universal compassionate care to alleviate suffering in irreversible illness.

The author's wife faced cancer. Cancer was the nightmarish dragon of suffering that drove Mrs. Humphry to choose euthanasia. There was no mention in *Final Exit* that Mrs. Humphry had been offered palliative care. So one must ask, "Who walked Mrs. Humphry's way?"

If caregivers are able to "walk the patient's way" through the art and science of humanitarian care, pain management, and the services of palliation, perhaps terminally ill patients can better negotiate their choices and their experience at life's further shores.

The story of Geri comes to mind. Despite consultation and collaboration with experts in advanced cancer pain and the use of self-administered intravenous narcotics, Geri continued to suffer unremitting pain. She fell into that small and terribly unfortunate percentage of patients whose pain could not be relieved. Notwithstanding the pain she endured, Geri did not at any time consider or make a request for euthanasia. When a patient is close to death and she or he has reached the breaking point of human endurance, death becomes a welcome friend. Geri's death was quiet, dignified, and peaceful: "God had wrapped up her pain."[9]

At the time of writing this book, euthanasia and physician-assisted dying were legal only in a few countries, mostly in Europe, and most notably in the Netherlands. Canada was in transition, while in the United States, a small number of states have legalized this option following the lead and example of the state of Oregon.

In the Netherlands legalized euthanasia under strict medical control has existed for decades. Yet at the same time, the health care system in the Netherlands actively promotes palliative care, thus safeguarding the dignity and the values of humanity.

It is interesting to note that one of the outcomes of legalized euthanasia and assisted dying in the state of Oregon and the Netherlands has been to foster the endorsement and acceptance of compassionate palliative care for those who are terminally ill.

Palliative care has gained international recognition as a specialized branch of medicine with expertise in the management of advanced tumor pain and the care of the terminally ill. Still, the reality remains that countless terminally ill patients do not receive palliation. Despite knowledge and progress, vast numbers

---

9. See the chapter, *'Detached Compassion': Geraldine.*

of people in the United States and throughout the world have no access to pain management and palliative care services.

The Netherlands, while permitting euthanasia under strict conditions, has made a concerted effort to offer palliative care to all those who need it. By 2004, the Netherlands had already established "approximately one hundred inpatient hospices, and twenty-four-hour pain-control hotlines that provide immediate advice for physicians."[28] Pain clinics complement public health. Consultation and collaboration between hospice teams and physicians has become the accepted norm. In the Netherlands, compassionate palliative patient care services are fully integrated into the health care system.

In other jurisdictions, much remains to be done to address the curse of unattended suffering in critical illness. This is a timely issue as the population ages, and it's an issue that affects us all. Effective methods of pain control, and the availability of regulated, self-administered analgesics for seriously ill patients who require it, are key to providing hope beyond despair. Thankfully, public awareness of the need for quality patient care is leading to an increase in the provision of palliative services both within hospices and within patient homes.

Advance Health Care Directive: The Living Will

*"What is important, in a sense,
is not so much the degree of choice the patient in fact has,
but whether or not he feels instrumental in
affecting what happens to him."*[29]

—Richard Totman

Participation in the management of one's illness restores the hope that one is heard and understood. And the decision to receive or refuse treatment is the right of every patient.

The doctor's role is to recommend and give advice. But there are times when illness prevents a person from communicating their acceptance of medical treatment. Discussion with family members and significant others about medical treatment in the event of catastrophic illness is a decision that should be planned ahead and documented.

A living will, or advance health care directive, personal care directive, or physician's directive, represents a person's wishes should a life-threatening illness or accident render them incompetent and unable to consent to or reject medical treatment to prolong their life. The directive must be signed and dated by the person who is making the medical request. Also, the contents of the document must be discussed with the person's family doctor, because, in the event of unconsciousness, that doctor will guide future medical interventions.

The tragic circumstances of Terry Schiavo, whose suffering was prolonged by artificial means for fifteen years as she lay in a persistent vegetative state, is a distressing example of what can happen to an individual when no living will is in place. To this day, value judgments, beliefs, and opinions about hastening or preventing the death of the dying remain contentious. Beyond the ideological and religious judgments of outsiders, the living will codifies a person's individual wishes and has the potential of preventing an unhappy fate of unwanted medical intervention. It also spares loved ones from being forced to make potentially agonizing decisions at a time of distress.

Unfortunate and distressing cases like that of Terry Schiavo, and cases of unacceptable medical intervention and nonintervention in catastrophic illness and near-death events, prove once again the desperate need for humanistic, compassionate care at life's conclusion.

Neil's Palliative Passport to Freedom

Neil was admitted to palliative care with end-stage leukemia. He celebrated his forty-fifth birthday with his wife and Dunira's hospice team. His wife, Muriel, was his staunchest supporter and personal mentor. They were a close-knit family that included twin fifteen-year-old boys.

Neil's work as a forest ranger played a huge part in his love of nature and the great outdoors. But for Neil, nature's presence remained far outside the walls of Dunira hospice. And he yearned to be in nature's midst.

Neil's illness was rapid in its progression and Dunira was Neil's choice for palliative care. Yet despite his choice, he felt terribly confined until Dr. Daniel provided Neil with the means to regain some peace of mind.

During their first patient-family-team meeting, Neil spoke of his hunger for the great outdoors. With a plan already in mind, Neil described his motorized bicycle. His love of bikes reminded Dr. Daniel of another young man, Paul, the racing cyclist, who also loved bikes.[10]

Neil made a simple request for a short day pass to ride around in the rain on his motorized bike. Neil's request was not beyond the realm of possibility, but it required a plan.

Neil said, "I love the soft spring rain. Everything smells so fresh and earthy. Rain makes me feel alive. The sun just hurts my eyes and reminds me that I'm sick. Maybe it's a lot to ask, since I'm a patient here. But I just want to ride my bike down David Street. I don't want to hang around here waiting to die."

Dr. Daniel nodded his approval. "Neil, if you feel up to it, I see no reason why we shouldn't encourage your David Street excursion. Your motorized bike shouldn't deplete your energy."

Dr. Daniel continued, "But it would be wise for you to carry a letter of instructions from me. I'll write a letter with my medical directive should any mishaps occur on the streets outside."

Dr. Daniel's letter provided Neil with peace of mind and a passport to freedom.

With that passport tucked safely inside his yellow waterproof poncho, Neil set off on his trip down David Street. On

10. See the chapter, *Paul's Journey.*

his outings in the rain, Neil always carried Dr. Daniel's medical directive. The medical directive stated that Neil was terminally ill and, in the event of a collapse or an accident, he was to be taken by ambulance to Dunira Hospice. The medical instructions further specified that there was to be no cardiopulmonary resuscitation. This palliative passport to freedom meant that Neil could safely venture outside without any fear of unwanted medical intervention in the event of an incident. This gave Neil great peace of mind.

During that short spring season, cloudy weather and gentle showers often found Neil on David Street. Neil's safe return to Dunira Hospice from his short bicycle day trips left him relaxed and at peace.

Thankfully, there was never a need to use the medical directive inside Neil's poncho pocket. To the satisfaction of Neil and his wife, he experienced no mishaps on his early afternoon outings and thus avoided any paramedic intervention.

Neil died without pain at Dunira, his temporary home and place of refuge.

———

Patients who receive palliative home care sometimes attach a copy of their advance health care directive to the door of the refrigerator in their kitchen. My seriously ill daughter found peace of mind in this practice, knowing that in the event of a medical emergency, she had taken precautions against paramedic rescue and unwanted medical intervention.

Hope Beyond Despair:
Victims of Injury

A Portrait of Suffering

Who made this dragon of untamed force?
Fired in the kiln, shaped in potter's clay,
Intractable, you came forth.
Oh fierce and mighty foe
did the fiery furnace claim you and make you what you are?
You lurk and hide and stalk the place where pain is to be found.
And then with might and vigor you strike your many blows
that maim the human spirit and devour the human soul.
Cunning is the motive that makes your victim host.

Outpatient clinics for pain management exist in major cities around the world. These clinics offer services to patients who suffer chronic pain, social trauma, and loss of health and well-being. Outpatient pain clinics offer pain management, biofeedback, hypnotherapy, and supportive group therapy. Victims of traumatic accidents who experience unremitting pain are among those that participate in these outpatient clinics.

What follows is the story of a sailor and his companion, a ceramic dragon that symbolized the sailor's unremitting pain. Their dry-land mooring was at the pain clinic of their maritime hometown.

Mr. Sailor was forty-four years old. Following an onshore accident, he endured thirty-four trigger points of pain.

In its temporary location, Mr. Sailor's anchor lay buried on the shore. His inability to venture out to sea forced him to chart an alternative course. He attended the pain clinic for treatment modalities. He also joined the support group. During one of the meetings of the support group, he told the members, "I'm longing to take my wife out for a cruise. But I'll *never* sail my yacht again. I've lost strength in my shoulders and arms. And that physio hurts like hell!"

Someone in the group answered. "Hey, *never* is a mighty big word. That's your dragon speaking. If you want to neutralize that dragon's power, you've gotta find another word."

One of the doctors suggested to the sailor, "You could try hypnotherapy. It might help ease that constant pain of yours."

One day later, Mr. Sailor sat quietly in the big reclining chair in my office and began a conversation.

"The doc believes in hypnotherapy. He said it would relieve my pain. I was skeptical 'cause I don't know how it works. But I'm willing to try. The doc said there's nothing to fear 'cause hypnotherapy's self-induced. He said you'd help me try."

Mr. Sailor then pointed to the place where his pain was most severe, and said, "Please take my pain away."

I nodded and replied, "Let's try to reduce your pain to tolerable, manageable limits. What reduction should we aim for?"

The sailor mulled it over for a few seconds, then said, "Let's shoot for a thirty percent reduction."

And with that target in mind we gave our concentration to his urgent request.

During hypnotherapy, Mr. Sailor gave up his struggle and

preoccupation with constant pain. He named the fears that held him captive. Then he witnessed and felt the dragon's awesome pain shrink in size. The manifestation of this powerful intervention empowered the sailor. And in the process of deep concentration, he achieved an altered, relaxed state that was akin to "waking-dreaming." Mr. Sailor saw himself aboard his yacht and felt the soothing movement of a gentle, peaceful sea. Hypnotherapy hushed the chatter of his worried mind and released him from the tyranny of his fear.

Several months later, following his discharge from the pain clinic, Mr. Sailor returned once more. He placed a large cardboard box on top of my desk, and said, "I've recently returned from my cruise to Alaska. My wife accompanied me on the cruise."

"How did you manage?" I asked.

"I thought about it a lot," he replied. "Then I came up with a plan. I had an outboard motor fitted to my yacht. And that made our sailing possible."

Mr. Sailor opened the large box on my desk and as he removed its contents, he said, "Take this ceramic dragon. I've made it for you. Use him in your work. Tell your stories around him. Information about pain that never ends is in short supply. I'll always remember the stories we shared. Those stories gave me hope and helped me see the obstacles that stood in my way."

Mr. Sailor's ceramic dragon stood fourteen inches tall. Its fearsome looks and spine of jagged peaks befitted its name. The sailor had named the dragon "Intractable" and it represented Mr. Sailor's motif for pain.

With good intentions, Mr. Sailor repeated, "Tell your stories around this dragon. Those stories helped me see what stood in my way. They gave me hope."

For Mr. Sailor, the ceramic dragon was a metaphor and symbol of his meaningless suffering and unattended pain. When he asked me to use that dragon in my work, he was referring to the power of sharing our stories, the power of deep listening with an open nonjudgmental heart, and the power of meeting those who are suffering in that common ground of shared humanity. These simple acts of compassion, humility, and humanity lie at the heart of the philosophy of palliative care, and that philosophy is as valid for those at the end of life as it is for anyone who is suffering the dragon of unending pain.

"Stay, Breathe with Me"

*The negation of suffering in illness
constitutes a major concern for all of humanity.*

Poets and scholars write about the frailty of human life. The breath not taken is all that separates us from life and living. Yet in death, memories of our life remain. In the cycle of events that shape our lives, we face hardships of unwanted change. But in fellowship with one another, we endure and gain an understanding of ourselves and of others. In our journeys through illness and struggle with despair, we uncover meaning and gain hope. Restoration of the human spirit grows from the wisdom that our heroes share, their memories never forgotten.

The stories in this book lay bare the reality of unattended suffering in catastrophic illness. Awareness of suffering's stark reality promotes the need for change in how we care for the seriously ill. At its heart, this narrative of illness is an appeal for change within the health care system, an appeal to eliminate the artificial barriers that distance professional caregivers from their patients.

The anguished cry, *"Stay, breathe with me,"* is both a plea and metaphor for awareness, understanding, and compassion.

Compassionate palliative care counteracts helplessness and suffering in catastrophic illness. Palliative caregivers have learned to listen to their patients. And with empathy and understanding, they provide altruistic care. For terminally ill patients and their families, palliation is both a necessity and a universal human right.

Attitudes towards illness are rooted in antiquity, philosophy, and medicine. Today, medical knowledge of illness and disease is monumental. But sadly, the meaning of suffering has been obscured by the science of technology.

The medicine of today relieves physical pain, curtails infections with antibiotics, and replaces malfunctioning organs. Malignant tumors are surgically removed or treated with chemotherapy. The doctor identifies the presence of illness and orchestrates treatment towards a cure.

But in this laboratory of technology, the patients' thoughts and feelings are unheard and remain unseen. Yet it is those same thoughts and feelings that reveal the meaning and impact of illness on patients and provide key insights in relationships of care.

The relief of suffering in illness ought to be a key principle of health care.

But it is not always so.

The evocative film *Wit*, based on the 1999 Pulitzer Prize–winning play of the same name by Margaret Edson, reveals the impact of negated suffering in irreversible illness. This powerful drama lays bare the immorality and indignity of patient subjugation by a paternalistic system that is inhumane, a system that dishonors the basic principles of humanity.

In the opening scene of *Wit*, the heroine, Vivian Bearing, renowned scholar and philosopher, receives the news that she is critically ill. Her cancer is advanced and her recovery hangs in the balance. She learns that an experimental treatment on offer will enhance medical knowledge and may lead to a miraculous cure. Vivian consents to the treatment.

But in the pursuit of fact-finding research, Vivian becomes the object of experimentation that is harsh and demeaning. She is faced with the indignity of diagnostic procedures that she loathes. She endures a state of enforced isolation to eliminate her risk of infection. Vivian's once familiar world disappears. Her pain is unremitting, chaotic, and she states, "I am learning to suffer."[30]

Relief from pain and suffering is a basic human right that applies to every person in need of compassionate care. The human rights of Vivian Bearing are shamefully dishonored.

To turn one's back on compassionate caring is to disown one's humanity. Healers and caregivers are participants in a drama that seeks emancipation from suffering. But all too often in pursuit of cure, the essence of meaning is discounted and, without meaning, there is no understanding, no compassion.

Only by fully entering into the drama of illness—without research props, without medical jargon that is cloaked in mystery—can we acquire the intrinsic meaning of suffering. It is then that "We will continue to know people at their most mature, and their most courageous."[31]

———

There are many heroes in this book. Courageous patients and caregivers who grappled head-on with the dragon of suffering, combining knowledge with compassion in the tender art of care. This book honors the humanity of fellow travelers, kindred spirits on many journeys shared.

The story of Mr. Farmer showed how paternalism and institutional "custodial" care needlessly magnified patient suffering.

Mrs. Lambie did not fully benefit from palliation because,

believing that God had forsaken her, she refused to participate with her caregivers in the management of her care. Nonetheless, Dunira Hospice provided a safe and caring place for her remaining days.

Through the looking glass of illness, Geri's courage spoke of her indomitable spirit. Despite her ungoverned pain, she found meaning in her life. Like so many courageous patients, Geri wholeheartedly participated with her palliative team of caregivers. She reached out to them and they reached back.

John Steele's suffering revealed the harm caused when communications break down and misunderstandings abound. Seumas and his wife, Kathleen, made us aware of the tyranny of imposed medical "truths" and the need for benevolence and compassion in the give-and-take of care. Sofia taught the meaning of humility and altruistic family care.

Along the way, we encountered Meg and Jessie, who shared their independence, their passion, and their love of life. From Roberta we learned of the impact of negative labels on vulnerable patients. Harry and Mabel showed us how they rejected labels, embracing instead their reality with courage and simplicity.

In the telling of his story, Paul cast aside his victim self and embraced his doctor within. Angie followed in his wake, as she exercised her patient rights.

By reaching into Dora's chaotic hysteria, we found a way to build a bridge and reduce her fears. Neil showed us how a palliative passport protected him and gave him joy in precious bike rides on outings from the hospice. And we witnessed the comforting solace of music.

Violet's story revealed the impact of an uncaring marriage on serious illness and how supportive others could alleviate some of her anguish. Heather listened to her father's stories and regained the essence of herself.

Through the art of story, Stephen's teacher found a way to reach a troubled child. Young Abby found a soul mate in the form of an anatomical puppet and a special way to communicate with her caregivers.

As we journeyed with Mr. Tee and his family, we witnessed a team of professional caregivers embrace community resources to address the multidimensional aspects of suffering. And we saw how, just as one offers a hand to another in need, palliation lies at the heart of community.

Like so many injured people who experience intense ongoing pain, Mr. Sailor wondered: *Who will listen? Who will understand?* His story shows the healing power of acknowledging the dragon of another's suffering, and how palliative techniques that combine pain management with simple acts of compassion, humility, and humanity can bring relief to someone suffering unending pain. At its core, palliation is the art of care for anyone who needs it.

From Wayne, Olga, Maria, Brian, Jock, and the sea captain, we learned of the support, camaraderie, and altruism experienced among hospice patients, families, and staff. We witnessed a marriage, celebrations, shared sorrows, and pleas for help. And we experienced how palliative care provides safety and support for persons at the further shores of life.

The heroes of each of these stories left behind something both infinite and precious.

Stories reveal realities that challenge, capture, and invite inquiring minds to venture into places unknown, places where we fear to go. But these are places we need to go if we are to provide compassionate, humanitarian care.

Fellow travelers in pursuit of healing care take heed:

Listen to the patient's story and you may understand.
Listen to the patient's story and find meaning
to guide your healing hand.

When illness disrupts the order of our lives, there is an urgent need to be heard and understood. Yesterday's shaman, who listened and walked the patient's way, is as vital as today's medicine in the mitigation of pain and suffering. The patients and families in this book shared their stories with their caregivers. We, in listening, became a team. And we named our care *palliation*.

On our journey through illness, we witnessed acts of courage, we learned and we grieved, and we embraced the miracle of laughter, music, and unconditional care. The end of this journey is a new beginning, a new reality, one that draws wisdom from this narrative of illness. We can use what we have learned as a guide to improve the quality of care for vulnerable patients and their families.

So many times, I overheard patients say:

"Tell my family not to bring me their long faces. Those long faces make me scared."

"Tonight I want to sleep in the family room with my partner."

"I just need a cuddle."

"Please don't bring me all that food. I'd love to eat it. But it won't stay down."

"I need to see my dog. He's a big mutt. But I love him. I hope he hasn't forgotten me."

"I'd love a visit from my cat. I miss her *so* much."

"Bring in the photos of our grandchildren. And the snaps we took of the garden."

"Tell me about your day and everything that happened along the way."

Our heroes said good-bye, but they never went away. They left behind their *Book of Life* to guide us on our way.

For Patients

What you can do to empower yourself:

- Know your rights as a patient.[32] And do not be afraid to stand up for your rights.

- Prepare an advance health care directive (living will), make sure that those in your life know about it, and give a copy to your family doctor.

- Get invested and personally involved in the management of your illness to preserve your dignity and safeguard your right to participate in decisions that affect your life.

- Exercise your freedom of choice in decisions that affect your medical care.

- Choose a family doctor who will listen to your story.

- Discuss your health care options with your family doctor and ask about hospital treatment, hospice care, palliative home care, and respite family care.

- If necessary, appoint an advocate to act on your behalf. A member of your family, or a trusted friend, may represent your wishes regarding medical decisions and treatment interventions. Keep your doctor informed.

- Challenge archaic ideas about illness that promote patient submission and helpless dependence.

- Be informed about the where and the why of your care.

- Know about the medicine that brings you relief from pain.

- Seek information about patient and family support groups.

- Take advantage of those patient and family resources that meet your particular needs, such as legal aid, social services, pastoral care, and volunteer transportation services.

- Surround yourself with those that you hold dear and those who inspire cheerful thoughts.

- In your life review, specify your needs and share your big and little hopes with the important people in your life.

- If hospitalized, know what helps you to relax, whatever brings you joy, including humor, books, audio books, music, films, photographs, and so on.

- In the give-and-take of care, maintain contact with the outside world and stay in touch to retain your bonds with the community.

- Consider the healing effects of meditation and guided relaxation to bring you peace of mind.

- Take control and express your needs.

- Let it be known to family and friends that their look of gloom brings you down. Let them know when you can't eat the food they bring. Don't be afraid to tell them when you need a hug, a nap, or want to be left alone.

- Do whatever works best for you, ask for help, indulge yourself, and let yourself be known as the person that you are.

References

1. Health and Welfare Canada, Ministry of Supply and Services Canada. *Cancer Pain: A Monograph on the Management of Cancer Pain*. Ottawa, Canada: Catalog Number H 42-2/5-1984E, 1984.

2. Hippocrates, cited in Siegel, B.S., MD, *Love, Medicine, and Miracles*. New York: Harper and Row, 1988, p. 2.

3. Kettner, S., "Puppets Help Ease Kids' Cancer Fears." CBC News, Technology and Science, September 15, 2003. Available online at: http://www.cbc.ca/news/technology/patient-puppets-help-ease-kids-cancer-fears-1.357202.

4. Rockwell, N., and T. Rockwell. *Norman Rockwell, My Adventures as an Illustrator*, reissue edition. New York: Harry N. Abrams, 1988, p. 222.

5. Bluebond-Langner, M., *The Private Worlds of Dying Children*, second edition. Princeton, NJ: Princeton University Press, 1980, p. 135.

6. Ibid., p. 205.

7. Health and Welfare Canada, *Cancer Pain: A Monograph on the Management of Cancer Pain*, p. 6.

8. Frankl, V.E., *Man's Search for Meaning*. New York: Simon and Schuster, 1962, p. 12.

9. Rozovsky, L.E., *The Canadian Patient's Book of Rights: A Consumer's Guide to Canadian Health Law*. Toronto: Doubleday of Canada, 1994, p. 42. Note: American readers can refer to: http://missinglink.ucsf.edu/lm/ethics/Content%20Pages/fast_fact_tx_refusal.htm

10. Nikiforuk, A., *The Fourth Horseman: A Short History of Epidemics, Plagues, Famines, and Other Scourges*. Toronto: Penguin Viking, 1991, p. xv.

11. Pope, A., "An Essay on Criticism: Part 2." First published in 1709, lines 230, 253, and 254 excerpted here. The full text is available online at: http://www.gutenberg.org/files/7409/7409-h/7409-h.htm

12. Saunders, C., M. Baines, and R. Dunlop, *Living with Dying: A Guide to Palliative Care*, third edition. Oxford: Oxford University Press, 1995, p. 47.

13. Health and Welfare Canada, *Cancer Pain: A Monograph on the Management of Cancer Pain*, p. 9.

14. Ibid., p. 23.

15. Frankl, V.E., *Man's Search for Meaning*.

16. Saunders, C. et al., *Living with Dying: A Guide to Palliative Care*, p. 15.

17. Cassell, Dr. E.J., "The Nature of Suffering and the Goals of Medicine." *The New England Journal of Medicine,* 306 (11), March 18, 1982, p. 639.

18. Ibid., p. 639.

19. Allen, J., *As A Man Thinketh.* 1902. Available online at: http://james-allen.in1woord.nl/?text=as-a-man-thinketh.

20. Ibid.

21. Nightingale, F., *Notes on Nursing: What It Is and What It Is Not.* Available online at: http://www.gutenberg.org/files/17366/17366-h/17366-h.htm

22. Frye, M.E., "Do Not Stand at My Grave and Weep." Included in a memorial service for United States Spanish War veterans held in Portland in 1938. Available online at various poetry sites.

23. Broyard, A., *Intoxicated by My Illness and Other Writings on Life and Death.* New York: Ballantine Books, 1992, p. 50.

24. Koestenbaum, P., *Managing Anxiety.* Millbrae, CA: Celestial Arts, 1979, p. 28.

25. Ibid., p. 40.

26. Quill, T.E., MD, and M.P. Battin, PhD, Eds., *Physician-Assisted Dying: The Case for Palliative Care and Patient Choice.* Baltimore: The John Hopkins University Press, 2004, p. 32.

27. Thomasma, D.C., and Graber, G.C., *Euthanasia: Toward an Ethical Social Policy*, New York: Continuum, 1990.

28. Quill, T.E et al., *Physician-Assisted Dying: The Case for Palliative Care and Patient Choice*, p. 330.

29. Totman, R.G., *Social Causes of Illness*. New York: Pantheon Books, 1979, p. 213.

30. Edson, M., *Wit: A Play*, first edition. New York: Faber & Faber, 1999.

31. Saunders, C. et al., *Living with Dying: A Guide to Palliative Care*, p. 58.

32. For readers interested in patient rights in Canada, refer to: Rozovsky, L.E., *The Canadian Patient's Book of Rights: A Consumer's Guide to Canadian Health Law*, Toronto: Doubleday Canada Limited, 1994. For readers interested in patient rights in the United States refer to: National Institutes of Health, US National Library of Medicine, "Patient Rights," online at: http://www.nlm.nih.gov/medlineplus/patientrights.html.

With Gratitude

Just as life's lessons take time to be valued and endorsed, the meaning and intent of this book was slow to take shape. From infancy to maturity, the book was aided by ordinary folks, just like you and me. And so, to the men and women who touched my life with their generosity of spirit, I give my thanks.

To Dr. Rev. David Skelton, my spiritual guide and mentor, who breathed life into the philosophy and meaning of compassionate patient care, thank you for your wisdom and your humanity.

To the late Professor Jim Gripton, who invested his time to advance the pursuit of knowledge shared, I owe much to his teaching and his humanity.

I am indebted to Mademoiselle Arlette Grumbach, former *chef du service de l'humanisation des hôpitaux à l'Assistance Publique*, who shared the philosophy of palliative medicine in France and who arranged visits to three Parisian hospices, including meetings with professional caregivers.

To the doctors, nurses, and diverse palliative teams, who willingly give of themselves to comfort the sick, my deepest appreciation. You are the unsung heroes who bring compassion, humility, and humanity to the most vulnerable.

When my daughter Irene and I completed an early draft of this book, several agents, as well as the senior editor of a well-known British publisher, were keen to represent it. But economic times and the challenge of convincing "marketing" teams of the relevance of this topic defeated them. Ironically, in trying to champion this book, these early supporters confronted the same challenges revealed throughout these pages: a fear of openly discussing grief, suffering, illness, pain, and death. But the times are changing. More books on these subjects are reaching readers. More doctors, nurses, and patients are lifting the veil of secrecy and the mystery surrounding serious illness and the inadequacy of a health care system so focused on technology and cure that it has lost sight of the person who is ill. More voices are joining the chorus to bring compassion back into health care, thereby reviving the healing art of care. In the context of this rising tide, this book found its publisher, She Writes Press. I am grateful to Brooke Warner, her talented team, and the incisive, insightful editorial eye of Wayne E. Parrish. Thank you.

To my family for their loving support, you have my utmost gratitude and eternal love. To my late husband, Walter, who guided my steps on a journey shared and who, with generosity and patience, edited the first draft of this manuscript. To Ken, who in times of fear and crises offered a safe, strong harbor. To Al, whose quiet presence prevails. To Kiera, who brings music and laughter.

And to my writing collaborator and daughter, Irene, who inspired this mother-daughter endeavor, who never gave up, and who ensured that this book became *this* book.

Finally, I would like to express my deepest gratitude to the men, women, and children whose stories fill the pages of this book, stories that eradicate fear, solitude, and pain. Thank you.

About the Authors

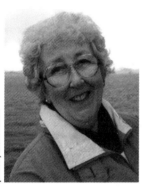

Helen Allison, RN, BA, BSW, MSW

Scottish highlander by birth, Helen studied nursing at Scotland's Dunbarton Joint Hospital, specializing in infectious disease during the deadly waves of tubercular meningitis, diphtheria, and whooping cough. Later she nursed at Scotland's Paisley Royal Alexander Infirmary.

After immigrating to Canada, Helen was invited to join as coordinator/head nurse at Canada's first palliative care unit, St. Boniface Hospital, Winnipeg. Throughout the decades, Helen nursed at other palliative care units across Canada. Later, she combined her mastery of nursing with medical social work in helping abused youth at the Children's Hospital.

During her long career as a palliative nurse and medical social worker, Helen pursued a person-centered approach to champion the ill and their families. Helen contributed to *Social Work Services as a Component of Palliative Care with Terminal Cancer Patients* (Haworth Press). Now, in *Stay, Breathe with Me: The Gift of Compassionate Medicine*, Helen shares her life's

photo by Irene Allison

learning that to ease suffering, the art of care must embody the wisdom of the patient.

Irene Allison

Irene, a former technical communicator, author and teacher, practiced for years in France, the United Kingdom, and Canada, and taught in the Writing and Publishing Program at

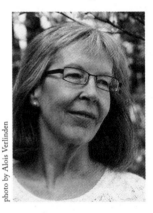

Simon Fraser University, a program from which she also graduated.

Today Irene writes stories about healing from the heart. She has a Post Graduate Certificate in Creative Writing from Humber College (Toronto) and has attended both the Arvon Institute (Scotland) and UBC's Booming Ground (Vancouver).

In *Stay, Breathe with Me: The Gift of Compassionate Medicine*, Irene is thrilled to join her mother in a growing international movement to bring heart into health care and compassion into our lives.

Visit Helen and Irene at: http://www.ireneallison.com

photo by Alois Verlinden

Dr. Rev. David Skelton, MB, BS, DM, MRCS, MRCP, MRCGP, FACP, M DIV.

A British-born geriatrician, Dr. Skelton graduated from the medical school of London's Westminster Hospital and was deeply affected by the work of Dame Cecily Saunders, founder of the modern hospice movement, with whom he attended rounds in the late 1960s at the original St. Christopher's Hospice.

Dr. Skelton played a crucial role in the early palliative care movement in Canada, creating the first hospice ward at St. Boniface Hospital, Winnipeg, in 1974, and later, a palliative care unit at the Edmonton General Hospital, Alberta.

Ordained as an Anglican priest in 1976, Dr. Skelton entered the Roman Catholic Church in 2012. In 1986, Dr. Skelton retired from the Edmonton Chair of Geriatric Medicine, but continued to work as a roving geriatrician in remote areas of Alberta and the Artic until 2010.

Throughout his lifelong contribution of caring for the ill and the elderly, Dr. Skelton was adored by his patients. A humanitarian of heart and humility, and blessed with a wonderful sense of humor, when he walked into the room, his very presence brought warmth and often laughter to those in need.

SELECTED TITLES FROM SHE WRITES PRESS

She Writes Press is an independent publishing company founded to serve women writers everywhere. Visit us at www.shewritespress.com.

From Sun to Sun: A Hospice Nurse's Reflection on the Art of Dying by Nina Angela McKissock. $16.95, 978-1-63152-808-8. Weary from the fear people have of talking about the process of dying and death, a highly experienced registered nurse takes the reader into the world of twenty-one of her beloved patients as they prepare to leave this earth.

Think Better. Live Better. 5 Steps to Create the Life You Deserve by Francine Huss. $16.95, 978-1-938314-66-7. With the help of this guide, readers will learn to cultivate more creative thoughts, realign their mindset, and gain a new perspective on life.

The Vitamin Solution: Two Doctors Clear the Confusion about Vitamins and Your Health by Dr. Romy Block and Dr. Arielle Levitan. $17.95, 978-1-63152-014-3. Drs. Romy Block and Arielle Levitan cut through all of the conflicting data about vitamins to provide readers with a concise, medically sound approach to vitamin use as a means of feeling better and enhancing health.

Beautiful Affliction: A Memoir by Lene Fogelberg. $16.95, 978-1-63152-985-6. The true story of a young woman's struggle to raise a family while her body slowly deteriorates as the result of an undetected fatal heart disease.

Green Nails and Other Acts of Rebellion: Life After Loss by Elaine Soloway. $16.95, 978-1-63152-919-1. An honest, often humorous account of the joys and pains of caregiving for a loved one with a debilitating illness.